TUMOURS, LYMPHOMAS AND SELECTED PARAPROTEINAEMIAS

Other titles in the *New Clinical Applications* Series:

Dermatology (Series Editor Dr J.L. Verbov)
Dermatological Surgery
Superficial Fungal Infections
Talking Points in Dermatology - I
Treatment in Dermatology
Current Concepts in Contact Dermatitis
Talking Points in Dermatology - II

Cardiology (Series Editor Dr D. Longmore)
Cardiology Screening

Rheumatology (Series Editors Dr J. J. Calabro and Dr W. Carson Dick)
Ankylosing Spondylitis
Infections and Arthritis

Nephrology (Series Editor Dr G.R.D. Catto)
Continuous Ambulatory Peritoneal Dialysis
Management of Renal Hypertension
Chronic Renal Failure
Calculus Disease
Pregnancy and Renal Disorders
Multisystem Diseases
Glomerulonephritis I
Glomerulonephritis II

NEW
CLINICAL
APPLICATIONS
DERMATOLOGY

TUMOURS, LYMPHOMAS AND SELECTED PARAPROTEINAEMIAS

Editor

JULIAN L. VERBOV

JP, MD, FRCP, FIBiol

Consultant Dermatologist,
Royal Liverpool Hospital,
Liverpool, UK

KLUWER ACADEMIC PUBLISHERS
DORDRECHT / BOSTON / LONDON

Distributors

---

for the United States and Canada: Kluwer Academic Publishers, PO Box 358, Accord Station, Hingham, MA 02018-0358, USA
for all other countries: Kluwer Academic Publishers Group, Distribution Center, PO Box 322, 3300 AH Dordrecht, The Netherlands

British Library Cataloguing in Publication Data

Tumours, lymphomas and selected paraproteinaemias.
1. Man. Skin. Cancer
I. Verbov, Julian II. Series
616.99'477

ISBN-13: 978-94-010-7683-8 e-ISBN-13: 978-94-009-2623-3
DOI: 10.1007/978-94-009-2623-3

Library of Congress Cataloging in Publication Data

Tumours, lymphomas, and selected paraproteinaemias/editor, Julian L. Verbov.
p. cm. — (New clinical applications. Dermatology)
Includes bibliographies and index.

1. Skin—Tumours. 2. Melanoma. 3. Lymphomas. 4. Paraproteinemia.
I. Verbov, Julian. II. Series.
[DNLM: 1. Skin Neoplasms. WR 500 T925]
RC280.S5T87 1988
616.99'477—dc 19
DNLM/DLC
for Library of Congress

Softcover reprint of the hardcover 1st edition 1988

Published in the United Kingdom by Kluwer Academic Publishers, PO Box 55, Lancaster, UK.

Kluwer Academic Publishers BV incorporates the publishing programmes of D. Reidel, Martinus Nijhoff, Dr W. Junk and MTP Press.

CONTENTS

LIST OF AUTHORS

Mr N.C. Davis, AO, MD, Hon DS, FRCS, FRACS, FACS
Consultant Surgeon
Chairman of Queensland Melanoma Project
Princess Alexandra Hospital
Brisbane
Queensland 4102
Australia

Dr M.C. Finan, MD
Senior Resident Associate
Department of Dermatology
Mayo Clinic and Mayo Foundation
Rochester
Minnesota 55905
USA

Dr A.W. Macfarlane, MRCP
Senior Registrar in Dermatology
Royal Liverpool Hospital
Prescot Street
Liverpool
L7 8XP

Dr N.P. Smith, MB, FRCP
Consultant Dermatologist
Skin Tumour Unit and Honorary Lecturer in Histopathology
The Institute of Dermatology
St John's Hospital for Diseases of the Skin
Lisle Street
Leicester Square
London
WC2H 7BJ

Dr M.F. Spittle, MSc, DMRT, FRCR
Consultant Radiotherapist and Oncologist
St John's Hospital for Diseases of the Skin
Lisle Street
Leicester Square
London
WC2H 7BJ
and Meyerstein Institue of Radiotherapy and Oncology
The Middlesex Hospital
London
W1N 8AA

Dr J.L. Verbov, MD, FRCP, FIBiol
Consultant Dermatologist
Royal Liverpool Hospital
Prescot Street
Liverpool
L7 8XP

Prof. R.K. Winkelmann, MD. PhD
Consultant , Department of Dermatology
(Mayo Clinic & Mayo Foundation)
Professor of Dermatology and of Anatomy
Mayo Medical School
Rochester
Minnesota 55905
USA

SERIES EDITOR'S FOREWORD

This, the seventh volume in the New Clinical Applications Series, has an international flavour, with contributions from Australia (Mr N.C. Davis), Great Britain (Drs A.W. Macfarlane, N.C. Smith, M.F. Spittle, J.L.Verbov), and USA (Dr M.C. Finan and Professor R.K. Winkelmann).

Dr Smith discusses some common skin tumours with his characteristic informative clarity. It is appropriate that an authority such as Mr Davis should discuss a tumour that has a particularly high incidence in his own country. Dr Spittle is a recognized authority on lymphomas and she writes succinctly on their management. Dr Finan and Professor Winkelmann have extensive experience of the rare condition, necrobiotic xanthogranuloma, and Drs Macfarlane and Verbov have been involved in the management of many patients with scleromyxoedema.

I am very pleased to have had the opportunity of working with the contributors and thank them most sincerely for their efforts.

I hope that this volume will interest dermatologists, oncologists, pathologists, radiotherapists and surgeons.

JULIAN VERBOV

ABOUT THE EDITOR

Dr Julian Verbov is Consultant Dermatologist to Liverpool Health Authority and Clinical Lecturer in Dermatology at the University of Liverpool.

He is a member of the British Association of Dermatologists, representing the British Society for Paediatric Dermatology on its Executive Committee. He is a Committee Member of the North of England Dermatological Society, and Editor of its *Proceedings*.

He is a Fellow of the Zoological Society of London and a Member of the Society of Authors. He is a popular national and international speaker and author of more than 200 publications.

His special interests include paediatric dermatology, inherited disorders, dermatoglyphics, pruritus ani, therapeutics, drug abuse and medical humour. He organizes the British Postgraduate Course in Paediatric Dermatology and is a Member of the Editorial Board of *Clinical and Experimental Dermatology*.

1

THE DIAGNOSIS AND MANAGEMENT OF COMMON SKIN TUMOURS

N. P. SMITH

INTRODUCTION

The skin is a complex organ derived embryologically from many different ectodermal and mesodermal structures. As well as the stratified squamous epithelium of the true epidermis, there are glandular structures, blood and lymphatic vessels, connective tissue, fat, melanocytes, Langerhans cells and numerous fixed tissue and circulating inflammatory cells, which can all on occasions produce skin tumours. The aetiology of these lesions depends on genetic as well as environmental factors. It is well known that some families are prone to develop malignant melanoma more frequently than the general population[1]. Other epithelial-derived tumours of the skin that may be familial include pilar cysts and some of the adnexal tumours such as cylindroma and trichoepithelioma[2]. Genetic defects in the ability to repair DNA damage satisfactorily are an important cause of the development of cutaneous tumours in xeroderma pigmentosum[3], and it is well known that individuals with a fair skin, red hair and a freckling tendency are at an increased risk of developing both epithelial and melanocytic malignant tumours. The basal cell naevus syndrome[4] is another example of an inherited condition in which there is a genetic predisposition to the development of basal cell epitheliomas in addition to many other cutaneous and non-cutaneous abnormalities.

Of the external and environmental factors that may be important in the aetiology of skin tumours, by far the most important is that of radiant energy. The commonest form of this to which we are all exposed is ultraviolet light. There is a clear association between chronic cumulative exposure to ultraviolet light and the incidence of certain epidermal tumours, such as basal cell carcinoma and squamous cell carcinoma. The relationship of the incidence of melanoma to exposure to ultraviolet light is more complicated. Malignant melanoma is not particularly common in outdoor workers, but there is some evidence to suggest that the development of malignant melanoma may be related to relatively short periods of exposure to high-intensity ultraviolet light[5]. Other forms of radiant energy, including X-rays and radiant heat, may also predispose the individual to the development of malignant skin tumours. Epithelial tumours of the scalp are not uncommon in patients who many years previously had radiotherapy to the scalp for treatment of tinea capitis.

Certain chemicals, both taken internally and acting externally as skin irritants, can be associated with the development of skin neoplasms. The increased incidence of Bowen's disease and epithelial tumours in patients who have ingested arsenic is well known. External irritants such as soot, tar products and mineral oils are also predisposing factors in certain occupations to the development of epidermal cancer and pre-cancer, although the classical chimney sweep's scrotal carcinoma is a rarity these days! The diagnosis and management of malignant melanoma and lymphoma are considered elsewhere in this volume (Chapters 2 and 3). I will confine my discussion to the diagnosis and management of relatively common lesions derived from the epidermis.

NAEVOID AND BENIGN PROLIFERATIONS OF THE EPIDERMIS

Epidermal naevus

Epidermal naevi are hyperplastic proliferations or hamartomas of squamous epithelium and sometimes other associated cutaneous structures, that are usually either present at birth or arise during childhood.

Clinical features

Epidermal naevi may occur anywhere on the body but are particularly common on the head and neck area. They usually have a warty or irregular surface and are often arranged in a linear or zosteriform fashion (Figure 1.1). The majority of lesions are under 5 cm in length, but widespread lesions are also seen. The variant naevus unius lateris is confined to one side of the body and may be extensive and pigmented.

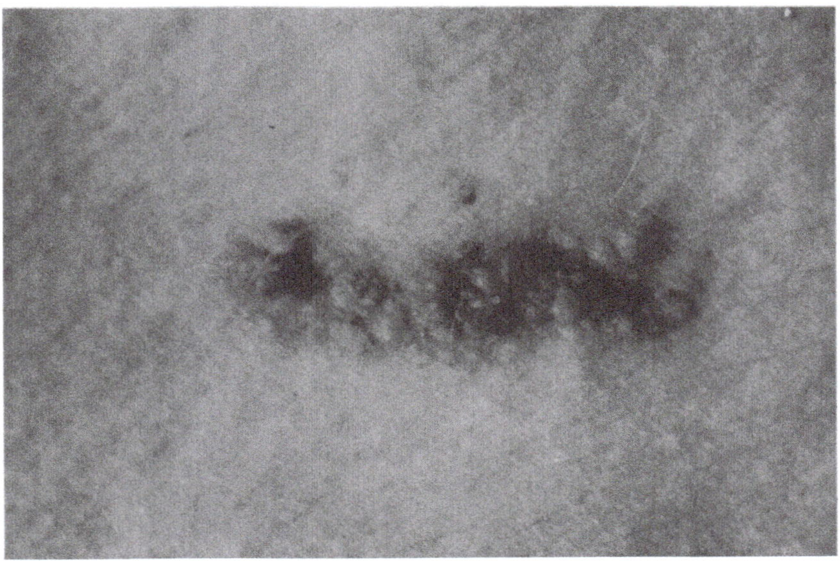

FIGURE 1.1 Linear warty epidermal naevus on the trunk

Naevus sebaceus (Figure 1.2) is a relatively common form of epidermal naevus, frequently affecting the scalp, that shows histological features of sebaceous gland hyperplasia as well as the presence of hyperplastic or deformed sweat gland structures. Sebaceous naevi (sometimes termed organoid naevi) are often relatively inconspicuous at birth, becoming larger and more obvious around the time of puberty, when patients with such lesions frequently seek advice for the first time. The incidence of the development within sebaceous naevi of other cutaneous tumours (particularly basal cell epithelioma and syringocystadenoma papilliferum) has probably been exaggerated; the chance of a malignant neoplasm developing is probably less than 15%[6].

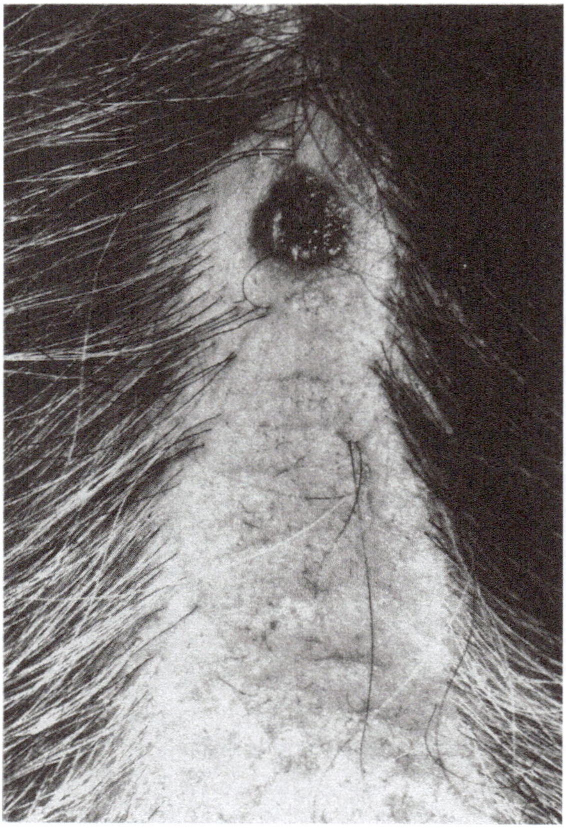

FIGURE 1.2 Naevus sebaceus of the scalp. A basal cell epithelioma has developed at one end of the lesion

One variety of naevus known as *inflammatory linear verrucous epidermal naevus* (ILVEN)[7] or *dermatitic naevus*[8] commonly affects the limbs, and because of its clinical appearance, often resembling psoriasis or eczema and the symptom of itching, may be misdiagnosed as an inflammatory condition. The linear configuration of these naevi, the history of persistence since birth or early childhood, and the absence of clinical evidence of inflammatory disease elsewhere, should help in making the correct diagnosis (Figure 1.3).

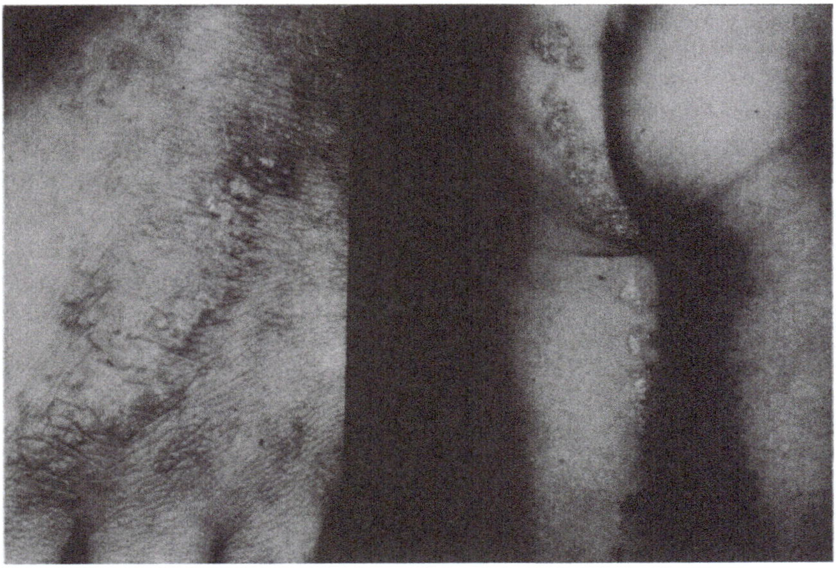

FIGURE 1.3 Inflammatory linear verrucous epidermal naevus (ILVEN) affecting the dorsum of the left hand and back of the left leg

Becker's naevus is a fairly common pigmented lesion, more common in males than females and tending, unlike many epidermal naevi, to develop in the second or third decade. The lesion varies in size and has irregular but well-defined borders and usually exhibits some degree of hypertrichosis.

It should be mentioned that, in some individuals, epidermal naevi may be associated with disorders of other organs (epidermal naevus syndrome)[9]. Lesions of the eye (lipodermoids, subconjunctival haemorrhages and colobomas), skeletal deformities (bone cysts, kyphoscoliosis, dental and rib abnormalities) and involvement of the central nervous system have all been reported. Large systematized epidermal naevi, especially those affecting the head and neck area are most likely to be associated with disorders of other organs.

Histology

The histopathology of simple epidermal naevi consists of varying degrees of hyperkeratosis, irregular acanthosis and papillomatosis. Hyperplastic or hamartomatous malformations of other cutaneous structures may be present in more complex naevi, including naevus sebaceous and Becker's naevus. The dermatitic naevus (ILVEN) shows histological features of psoriasiform inflammation in addition to simple epidermal hyperplasia. Other naevi may show the histological appearances of epidermolytic hyperkeratosis, Darier's disease[10], porokeratosis or comedo-like changes[11].

Management

Small epidermal naevi are most appropriately treated by surgical removal if required. Most authorities recommend excision of sebaceous naevi because of the small risk of the development of malignant change. Apart from formal surgery, other destructive techniques such as cryotherapy and dermabrasion[12] have been used with varying degrees of success. Drug therapy has little role in the management of epidermal naevi, although topical keratolytics and antimicrobial preparations may produce symptomatic improvement in some lesions and systemic retinoids[13] have been described as having a useful effect in others. The presence of associated underlying lesions in other organs (epidermal naevus syndrome) should always be considered, especially with large lesions.

Seborrhoeic wart (Syn. seborrhoeic keratosis, basal cell papilloma)

This lesion is one of the commonest benign epidermal neoplasms with an incidence that increases from the fourth to the seventh decades of life. Genetic factors may play a part in its development.

Clinical features (Figures 1.4 and 1.5)

Seborrhoeic warts may occur anywhere on the hair-bearing skin, but they are particularly common on the trunk and sites exposed to sun. Individual lesions vary in size from a few millimetres to several centimetres and often have a 'stuck-on' appearance. The surface of seborrhoeic warts may be flat and smooth, or, more commonly, verrucous and uneven. Though commonly brown in colour, they may vary from dull yellow or flesh-coloured to black. Very dark lesions may be clinically misdiagnosed as malignant melanoma. An individual may have a few lesions or several hundred. The sudden eruption of multiple lesions over a short period of time may be associated with an acute inflammatory process in the skin such as erythrodermic eczema (Murray Williams warts)[14] or, especially if accompanied by itching, the presence of internal malignancy (the sign of Leser-Trélat)[15] . The lesions known as stucco keratoses[16] and dermatosis papulosa nigra[17] can be considered particular variants of seborrhoeic warts.

Histology

Microscopically, seborrhoeic warts are basal cell papillomas associated with varying degrees of hyperkeratosis. The basaloid cells composing the bulk of the tumour probably represent immature and undifferentiated keratinocytes. These basaloid cells may contain melanin pigment. Lesions may be flat or raised and predominantly acanthotic seborrhoeic warts differ in their histological appearance from predominantly hyperkeratotic lesions (Figures 1.4 and 1.5). Keratinous cysts are frequently seen within these tumours and inflammation secondary to external trauma or irritation may produce foci of keratinocytes with more abundant cytoplasm closely resembling normal epidermal cells. These 'whorled' foci of paler and larger keratinocytes within areas of basaloid cells are sometimes known as squamous eddies.

Management

Seborrhoeic warts are normally an essentially cosmetic problem. The superficial nature of the lesions makes them suitable for removal by simple curettage and electrodesiccation. Other surgical modalities, such as cryotherapy, also have their advocates.

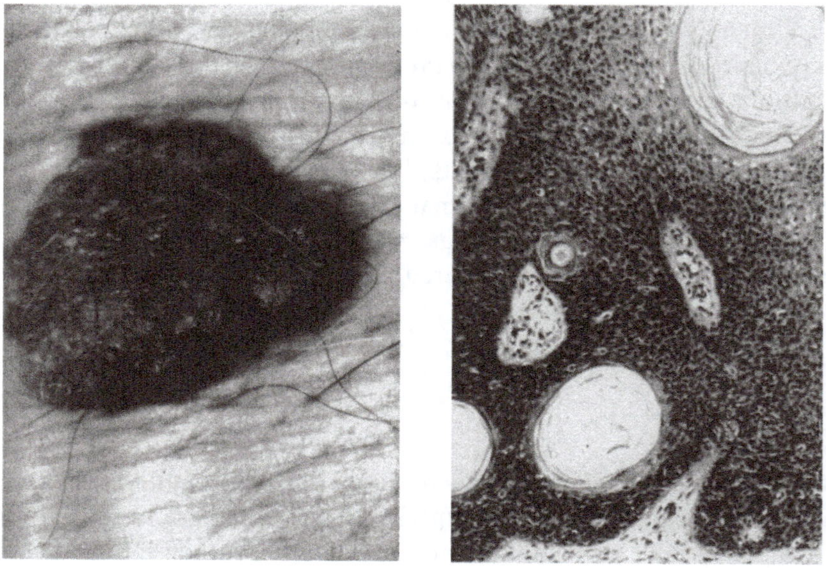

FIGURE 1.4 Acanthotic seborrhoeic wart with corresponding histology composed predominantly of small basaloid epithelial cells

Degos' acanthoma (Syn. clear cell acanthoma)

This lesion is a relatively uncommon epidermal tumour composed histologically of clear cells containing glycogen.

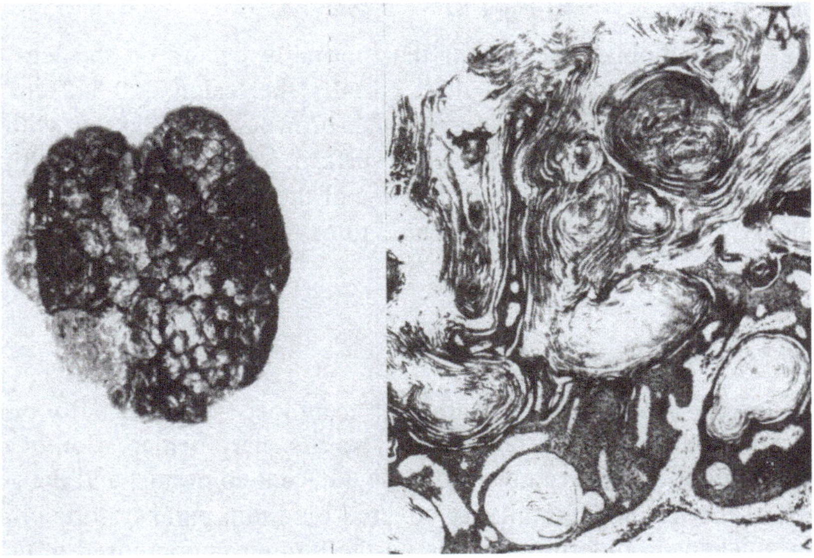

FIGURE 1.5 Hyperkeratotic seborrhoeic wart. Histology shows gross thickening of the stratum corneum

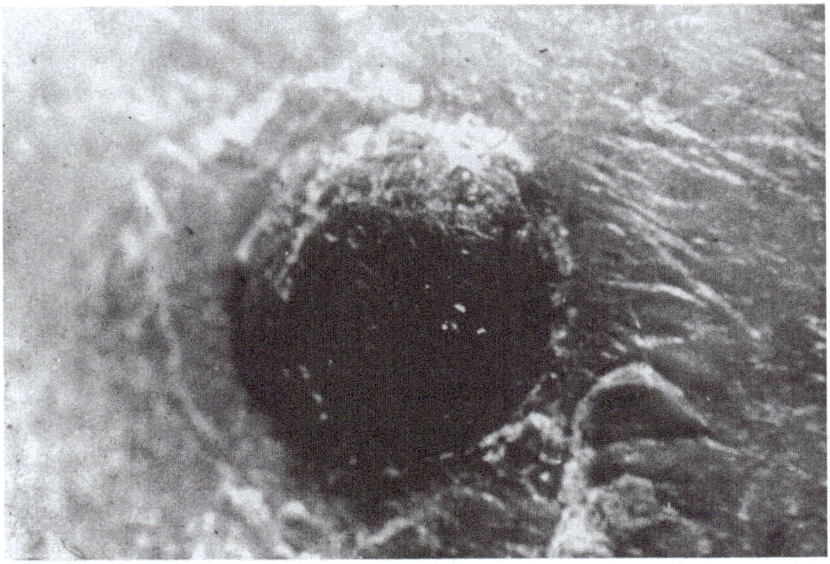

FIGURE 1.6 Degos' acanthoma. Typical raised symmetrical lesion with eroded surface

Clinical features[18] (Figure 1.6)

Degos' acanthoma is a tumour that normally occurs on the legs of middle-aged or elderly patients. Usually the lesion is 0.5–2 cm in size, a circumscribed, raised, reddish-brown nodule, often with a moist, glistening or slightly scaly surface. Occasionally, multiple lesions have been reported and, in some of these cases, ichthyosis[19] and other dry, scaly dermatoses appeared to be a predisposing factor.

Histology[19]

The lesions show variable degrees of acanthosis; this is usually more marked in the centre of the lesion. There is sharp demarcation of the lateral borders of the tumour from the adjacent epidermis and the surface of the lesion is commonly covered by a thin parakeratotic crust. The thickened epidermis making up the tumour is composed of cells with light-staining nuclei and abundant clear cytoplasm. The presence of glycogen in these cells can be demonstrated by the use of the periodic-acid-Schiff (PAS) staining technique. Other histological features that may be present in these lesions are the presence of inflammatory cells (predominantly neutrophil polymorphs) within the acanthotic epithelium and sweat gland hyperplasia in the underlying dermis.

Management

Simple excision is the treatment of choice for such lesions.

Keratoacanthoma (Syn. molluscum sebaceum)

Keratoacanthoma is a benign self-healing tumour that grows rapidly to form a crateriform nodule with a keratotic centre and which, after several weeks or months, regresses spontaneously to leave a depressed and irregular scar. In its early stages, there may be histological confusion with squamous cell carcinoma.

Clinical features[20] (Figure 1.7)

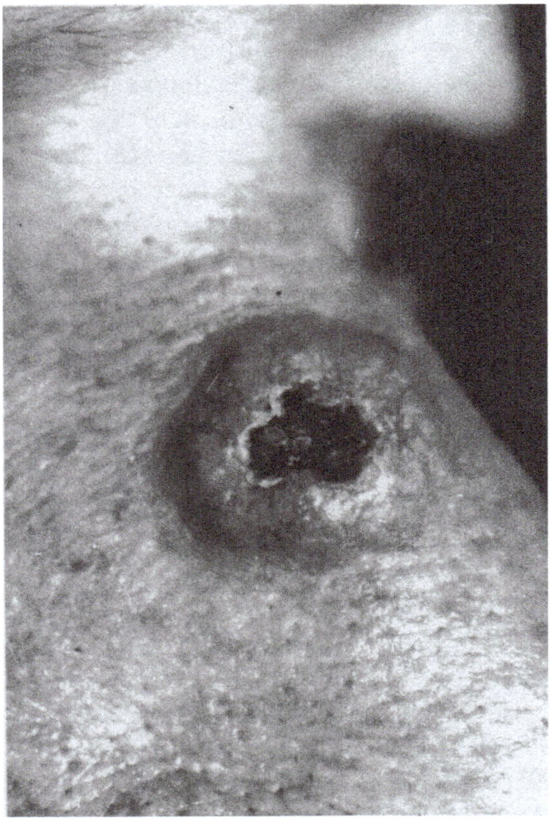

FIGURE 1.7 Keratoacanthoma. Symmetrical domed nodule with central keratin-filled core

Keratoacanthomas may occur on practically any body site, although the most commonly affected sites are those of the central face, ears and dorsal surfaces of the upper limbs. Unusual sites occasionally involved by keratoacanthomas include the mucous membranes of the mouth and the nail bed[21]. Men are affected twice as commonly as women and the peak incidence of the condition is in the fourth to sixth decade of life. Keratoacanthomas may result from faulty pilosebaceous follicle differentiation, and chronic solar damage and minor local trauma have been described as predisposing factors. Lesions have occurred as complications of xeroderma pigmentosum and have been associated with internal carcinoma in Torre's syndrome. The question whether a keratoacanthoma can ever behave in a truly malignant way is very controversial. Although aggressive forms of lesion[22] and metastasizing examples of keratoacanthoma[23] have been described, it is difficult to be sure that some such lesions are not better classified as forms of squamous cell carcinoma.

Several variants of keratoacanthoma have been described. Giant lesions that continue to enlarge for many months have been recognized. Keratoacanthoma centrifugum marginatum[24] is a rare variant that is characterized by a lesion that continues to extend peripherally for several years, while at the same time healing behind the advancing edge, giving rise to a large area of scarring.

Multiple keratoacanthomas may occur in association with local skin disease, including eczema, psoriasis, lupus erythematosus and follicular mucinosis. A rare condition described by Winkelmann and Brown[25] is that of generalized eruptive keratoacanthoma. In this condition, the onset is sudden, with a profuse eruption of tiny individual lesions becoming confluent on the face and central parts of the body. Ectropion and narrowing of the mouth may occur; pruritus is a prominent symptom; and involvement of oral and laryngeal mucosa has been described.

Although the lesions described by Ferguson-Smith as multiple self-healing squamous epithelioma[26] have some characteristics in common with keratoacanthoma, there are also clinical and histological differences. This condition is probably inherited as an autosomal dominant; it affects men more commonly than women; and the mean age of onset is in the mid-twenties. Multiple acneiform lesions occur predominantly on exposed sites and gradually heal to leave irregular and unsightly scars. The histology of lesions may be impossible to differentiate from squamous cell carcinoma but the lesions never metastasize.

Histology

The histological appearances of keratoacanthoma depend on the phase of growth of the lesion when biopsied. It is essential for diagnosis to have a representative biopsy of reasonable size, which ideally should be taken through the whole lesion and include normal surrounding skin. A mature keratoacanthoma is composed of a symmetrical mass of proliferating and keratinizing squamous epithelium with the central and upper portions of the lesion filled by keratinous material. The periphery of the lesion is formed by well-differentiated squamous epithelium and a characteristic feature is the presence of thinned and stretched epithelium extending over the sides of the tumour to form 'shoulders'. Mitotic figures, atypical keratinocytes and evidence of premature keratinization are seen in keratoacanthoma, but these features are more prominent at the actively growing deep and peripheral margins of the lesion. A dense, predominantly mononuclear cell, inflammatory cell infiltrate is commonly present deep to and around the epithelial tumour. The most important problem in differential diagnosis is the separation of keratoacanthoma from squamous cell carcinoma. As has been mentioned, this may be difficult with the lesions of Ferguson-Smith disease, but a typical

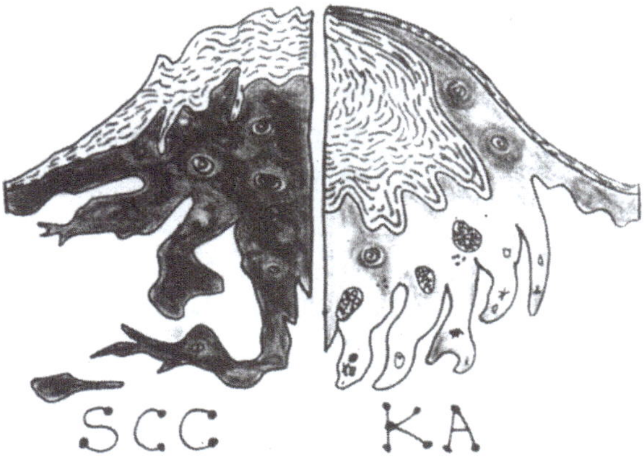

FIGURE 1.8 Diagrammatic summary of different histological features seen in a typical squamous cell carcinoma (on left) and keratoacanthoma (on right). (See text for details)

keratoacanthoma differs from a squamous cell epithelioma in several respects; these are summarised in Figure 1.8. The histological features favouring a diagnosis of keratoacanthoma include bilateral symmetry, an expansile growth pattern, and the presence of thin epithelial 'shoulders' surrounding the central horny plug. Mitotic figures and atypical tumour cells should be confined to growing margins of the lesion and the presence of intraepithelial neutrophil polymorph microabcesses is said to be a pointer towards the diagnosis of keratoacanthoma rather than squamous cell carcinoma. In the late stages of keratoacanthoma the histology is frequently non-diagnostic, often amounting to little more than an area of irregular squamous epithelium with underling dermal fibrosis.

Management

Formal surgical excision of keratoacanthoma leads to the best cure rate. The added advantage of this procedure is that one has the whole lesion for proper histopathological evaluation. Because of the exophytic nature of keratoacanthomas, the tumours are frequently treated by curettage and cautery. Recurrence may be seen following this procedure, but the majority of lesions heal satisfactorily. For multiple or giant lesions, various systemic drugs have been used including methotrexate and retinoids[27,28]. Intralesional bleomycin[29] and topical[30] and intralesional fluorouracil[31] have also been described as useful.

PREMALIGNANT EPIDERMAL LESIONS AND CARCINOMA *IN SITU*

Actinic keratosis (Syn. solar keratosis, senile keratosis)

Actinic keratoses are extremely common lesions that occur in the areas of the skin exposed to light and increase in frequency with age. Red-haired, blue-eyed and fair-skinned people, as well as those who never tan but burn easily in the sun, are at increased risk of developing keratoses. It is clear that exposure to ultraviolet light plays an important part in their development and it has been estimated that keratoses may be present in up to 50% of individuals aged 40 and over living in sunny climates such as that of Australia[32]. Squamous cell carcinoma may develop from actinic keratoses, but the risk of this occurring has probably been over-estimated in the past[32]. Lesions that are clinically and histologically similar to actinic keratoses may develop following exposure to tar and mineral oils and ionizing radiation, and in patients who have received arsenic.

Clinical features

The lesions most commonly occur on the face and backs of the hands, but may also be widespread on the forearms and upper trunk, depending on the extent and degree of exposure to sun over the years. Individual keratoses are pink, grey or brownish-red in colour and usually have some degree of surface scale (Figure 1.9). Larger lesions may resemble cutaneous lupus erythematosus. Variants of keratosis include a hypertrophic variety that may produce unusual

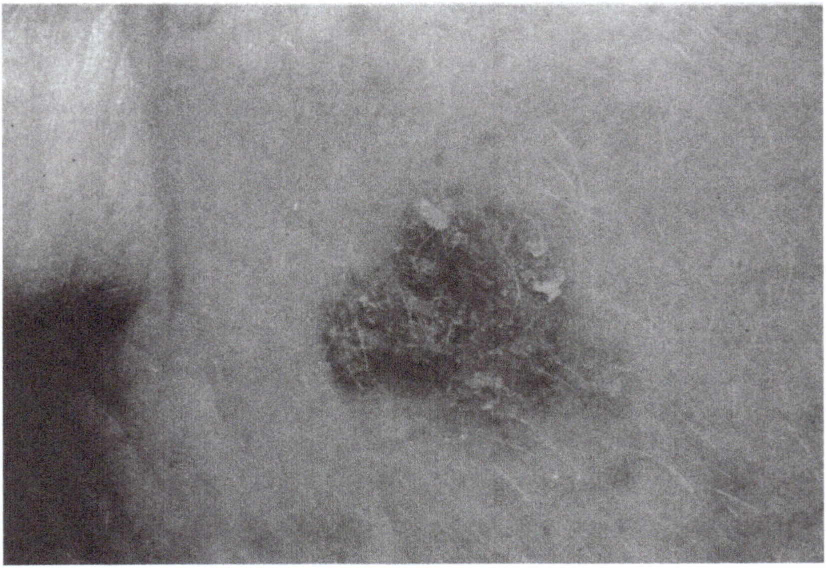

FIGURE 1.9 Actinic keratosis. Erythematous scaly plaque on sun-damaged skin of cheek

horn-like protuberances (cutaneous horn), atrophic and lichenoid keratoses[33], and a pigmented variety that may be mistaken for a flat seborrhoeic wart or lentigo maligna[34].

Histology[35]

The major histological feature is the presence of abnormal (dysplastic) squamous cells in the epidermis, particularly in the basal layers. Individual keratinocytes show cytological and nuclear atypia and evidence of premature or abnormal keratinization, and mitotic figures may be seen. The cells forming the epidermis also lose their normal relationship to one another and the regular, ordered appearance of the epidermis as a whole disappears (loss of polarity). The stratum corneum overlying the abnormal portions of epidermis normally shows parakeratosis. The dysplastic epidermal changes tend to be confined to the inter-adnexal epithelium, the epidermis immediately surrounding eccrine sweat ducts, and pilo-sebaceous follicles being

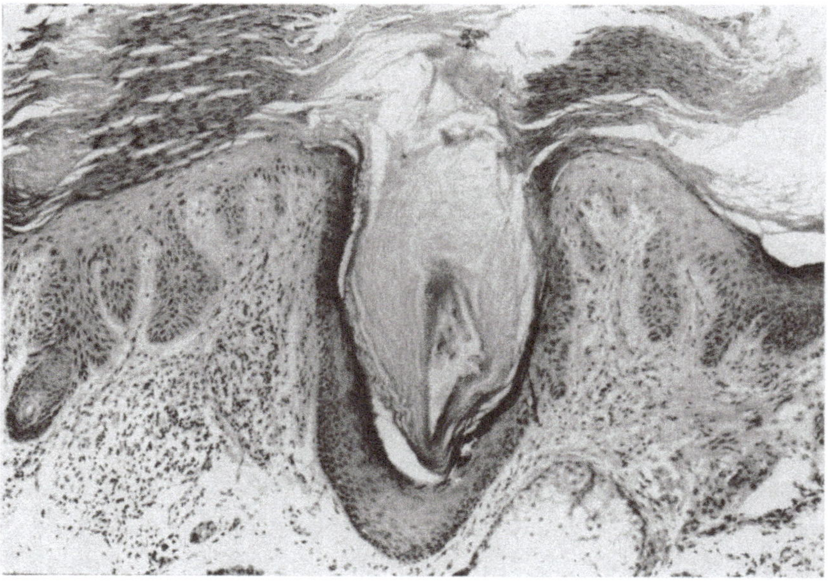

FIGURE 1.10 The typical histological features of an actinic keratosis. (See text)

preserved, with no cell atypia and overlying orthokeratosis (Figure 1.10). The degree of histological abnormality varies considerably from gross 'Bowenoid' dysplasia to very subtle changes in the lower layers of the epidermis. Hypertrophic, atrophic and lichenoid clinical varieties of keratoses show corresponding histological changes. The separation of individual keratinocytes from one another (acantholysis) is quite frequently seen in actinic keratoses. Dermal changes that are usually present include a chronic inflammatory mononuclear cell infiltrate immediately below the abnormal epithelium and a change in the appearance of dermal collagen known as solar elastosis. Many histological variants of actinic keratosis have been described, including large-cell acanthoma[36] and an epidermolytic variant[37].

Management

Individual lesions may be dealt with by curettage and cautery, cryosurgery or formal excision. Topical 5-fluorouracil normally used as a 5% ointment is effective in many patients. The ointment is applied twice daily for 2–4 weeks and causes local inflammation in the affected skin. It is important to warn the patient that this will occur, as the inflammatory change can be quite marked in some individuals. Some clinicians use a topical steroid preparation after the first signs of a reaction, to damp down the inflammatory episode. When the reaction has subsided, the actinic keratosis is found in most cases to have disappeared. The use of 5-fluorouracil ointment on sun-damaged skin that appears clinically normal can reveal the presence of further unsuspected keratoses. The success rate of the treatment of actinic keratoses by this method varies but is generally not quite as good as the surgically destructive treatments. Some success in the management of multiple keratoses has been claimed for oral etretinate[38]: a majority of patients studied over a four-month period showed a complete or partial response. In addition to specific therapeutic measures directed towards destruction of the keratoses themselves, it is of course essential to advise patients on the importance of avoiding excessive exposure to sun and on the appropriate use of sun-screens.

Bowen's disease

This is a form of epidermal carcinoma *in situ* that is less clearly related to exposure to sun than is actinic keratosis. It may be associated with the ingestion of trivalent inorganic arsenic compounds many years previously. Arsenic was given therapeutically for psoriasis, epilepsy and multiple sclerosis and was added to 'iron tonics' prescribed for anaemia. Bowen's disease is generally regarded as premalignant, an invasive squamous carcinoma arising in approximately 3–5% of patients[39]. It should be remembered that arsenic-related Bowen's disease is associated with visceral malignancy (especially carcinoma of the bronchus) in a number of individuals[40].

Clinical features (Figure 1.11)

Lesions of Bowen's disease may occur anywhere on the body, in areas exposed to light or not. They are pink-to-red, scaly, thickened, sharply circumscribed patches that may be up to several centimetres in size. Occasionally they may be heavily pigmented[41]. Clinically,

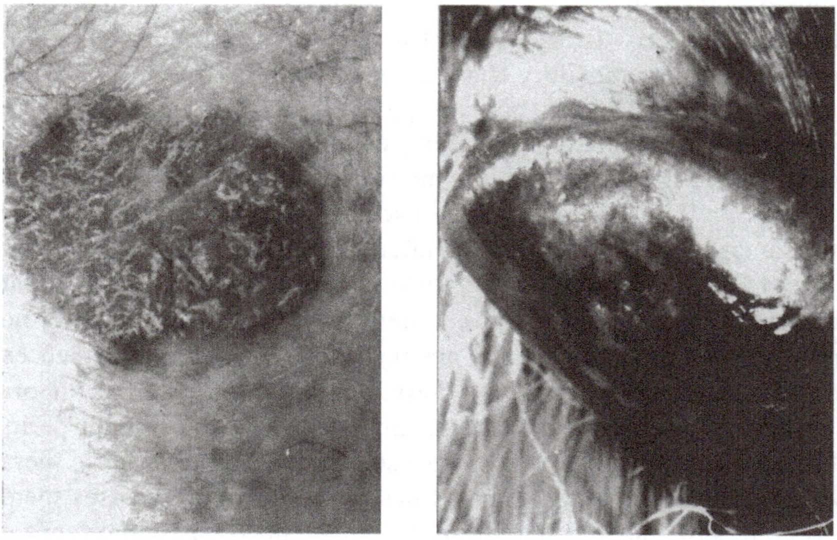

FIGURE 1.11 Plaque of Bowen's disease (on left) and erythroplasia of Queyrat affecting the glans penis (on right)

Bowen's disease may be misdiagnosed as inflammatory conditions such as psoriasis or discoid eczema, the superficial variety of basal cell epithelioma or actinic keratosis. Like actinic keratoses, lesions may be warty and hypertrophic, sometimes producing a cutaneous horn. When Bowen's disease affects the glans penis, the disorder is known as erythroplasia of Queyrat and has different clinical features from the condition seen elsewhere; the surface has an eroded or glazed appearance and the lesions are often bright red in colour. Another condition closely related to Bowen's disease is that of *Bowenoid papulosis (multicentric pigmented Bowen's disease of the genitalia)*[42]. The clinical lesions are flat or verrucous, often pigmented, papules occurring on the genital skin in young patients of both sexes (Figure 1.12). Clinically, the lesions may resemble viral or seborrhoeic warts and are frequently multiple. The histology may be indistinguishable from Bowen's disease itself, but progression of Bowenoid papulotic lesions to invasive squamous carcinoma rarely, if ever, occurs. Certain types of human papilloma virus have been suggested as a cause of at least a proportion of cases. There are many reports of lesions undergoing spontaneous remission.

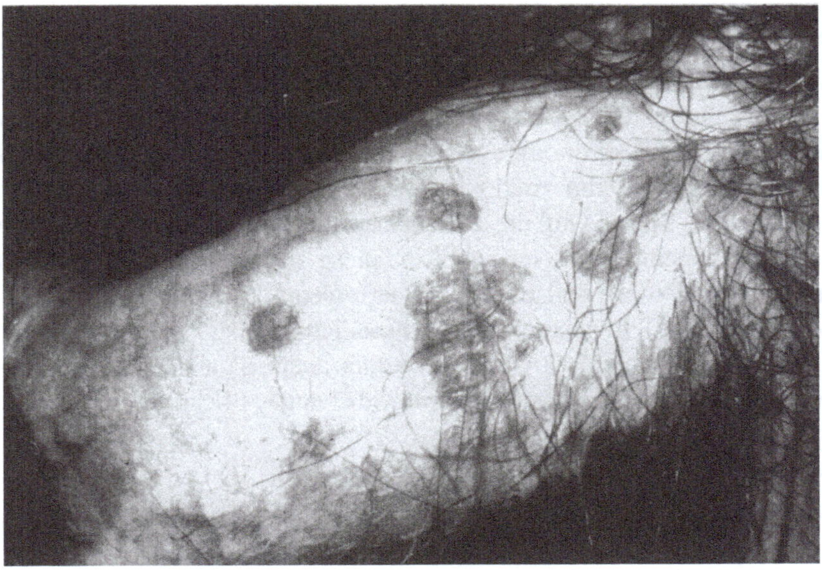

FIGURE 1.12 Lesions of Bowenoid papulosis on the shaft of the penis

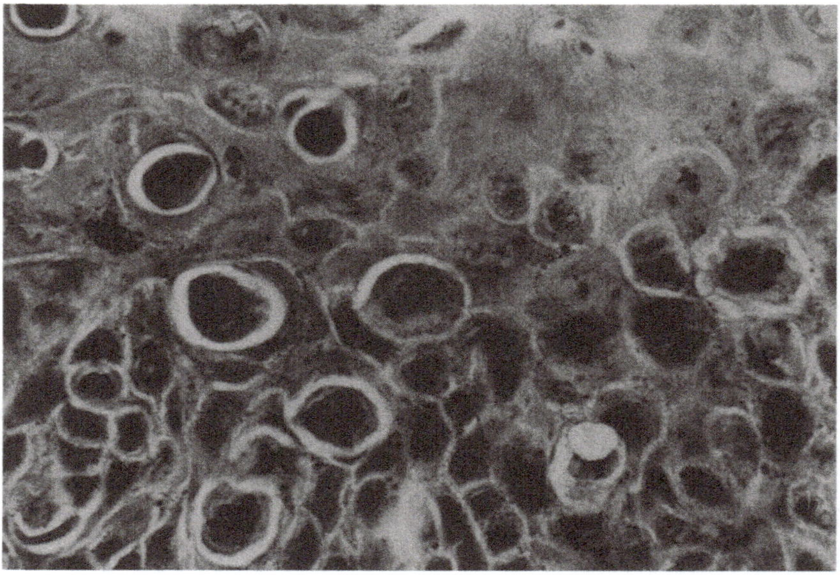

FIGURE 1.13 Keratinocyte atypia, mitotic figures and loss of polarity. The histological features of Bowen's disease

The histological features of Bowen's disease (Figure 1.13), erythroplasia of Queyrat and Bowenoid papulosis are those of carcinoma *in situ*. There is keratinocyte atypia and loss of polarity, and mitotic figures (including abnormal forms) may be present at all levels of the epithelium. Sparing of the adnexal epithelium, as occurs in actinic keratoses is sometimes seen, but in these situations a precise differentiation of Bowen's disease from a Bowenoid actinic keratosis may be impossible. In lesions of Bowenoid papulosis, histological features of seborrhoeic wart or condyloma acuminata may be superimposed upon the full-thickness dysplastic changes of carcinoma *in situ*.

Management

Surgical measures including cryotherapy are effective in treating lesions of Bowen's disease. Topical 5-fluorouracil ointment is also useful in many cases, but it should not be used if there is any clinical suspicion of the development of early invasive squamous cell carcinoma. Lesions of Bowenoid papulosis should be managed by conservative surgical procedures or even a 'wait-and-see' policy, as spontaneous resolution may occur in this condition. In Bowenoid papulosis, there is no indication for the aggressive surgery, such as radical vulvectomy, which has been carried out in some patients.

MALIGNANT EPIDERMAL TUMOURS

Basal cell epithelioma (Syn. basal cell carcinoma, basalioma)

Basal cell epithelioma is probably the most commonly occurring cutaneous malignant tumour worldwide. Its incidence is closely related to cumulative exposure to sunlight and it is therefore more common in older individuals and out-door workers, and in countries closest to the equator. The tumour is much more common in fair-skinned individuals who burn easily in the sun, particularly those of Celtic extraction; however, basal cell epithelioma has been described in most racial groups. Other factors predisposing to the development of this tumour include certain genetic disorders (xeroderma pigmentosum, basal cell naevus syndrome), immune suppression, arsenic ingestion, cutaneous irradiation and possibly local trauma such as burns and smallpox vaccination[43].

Although conventionally classified as a malignant tumour, basal cell epithelioma usually exhibits only slow local progressive growth, metastases occurring very rarely[44]. Of the relatively few cases of well-documented metastasizing basal cell epithelioma in the literature, most have been atypical lesions, often with a history of repeated and incomplete surgery or radiotherapy treatment[45]. The relatively benign biological course of these tumours makes the term epithelioma more appropriate than carcinoma.

Clinical features

As is the case with many common cutaneous lesions, the clinical presentation of basal cell carcinoma may be extremely variable. The

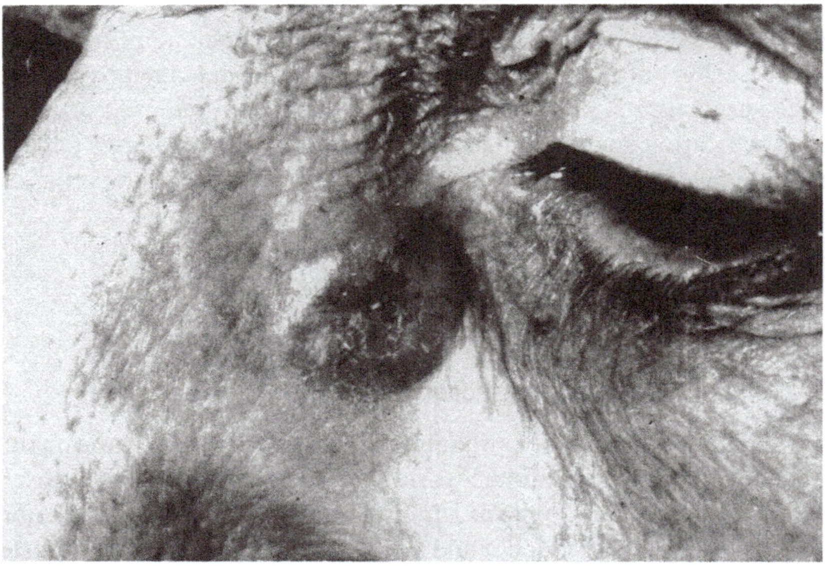

FIGURE 1.14 A typical papulonodular basal cell epithelioma

characteristic history is that of a slowly developing indurated area of skin on a site exposed to sun, which gradually increases in size to form a nodule, often with surface erosion or ulceration. Recurrent surface crusting and scab-formation is common. The tumour itself may have a translucent or 'pearly' quality and surface telangiectasia is sometimes seen. The lesion is firm to palpation and a well-defined edge is normally observed when the skin is stretched. Other features of sun-damage, such as solar elastosis, sebaceous hyperplasia and actinic keratoses, may be seen in the nearby skin. The papulonodular type of basal cell epithelioma described above (Figure 1.14) is the commonest, but other forms include cystic, pigmented, superficial and morphoeic varieties. The pigmented variety contains melanin and clinically lesions are not infrequently misdiagnosed as malignant melanomas or other melanocytic tumours. The superficial type of tumour (often erroneously called multifocal) usually consists of a flattish, pink-to-red, scaly plaque resembling Bowen's disease or even a patch of psoriasis or eczema. This variety of basal cell epithelioma is frequently multiple and affects sites of the body not exposed to sun, such as the trunk, more commonly than other varieties of the tumour. Distinction from Bowen's disease and inflammatory conditions of the skin may be made by stretching the skin, when a thread-like edge to the lesion may be seen sharply separating the tumour from the surrounding skin. Morphoeic basal cell epithelioma presents as an ill-defined, often whitish, sclerotic area of skin induration. This lesion has a bad reputation for recurrence following treatment, but this may simply reflect the difficulty in precise delineation of tumour margins both clinically and histologically.

Histology

Basal cell epithelioma is a tumour characterized by sheets, nests or strands of small basaloid cells with a relatively small amount of cytoplasm and a large oval nucleus. The cells at the peripheral portions of the tumour are often elongated and arranged in a palisade (Figure 1.15). Following normal fixation and embedding processes, it is

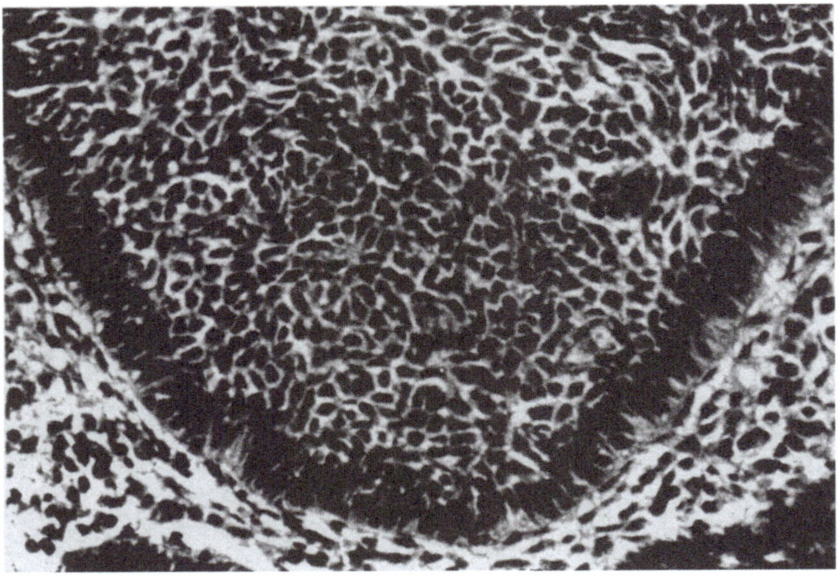

FIGURE 1.15 An island of basaloid tumour cells with peripheral palisading. The histology of part of a basal cell epithelioma

quite common for tumour islands to shrink away from the surrounding connective tissue, producing the so-called separation artefact. The great majority of basal cell epitheliomas are seen to be in continuity with either the epidermis or adnexal epithelium and most tumours are associated with a mucin-rich connective tissue stroma. Degeneration may sometimes occur within tumour islands, producing the histological cystic or adenoid variant of lesion. Melanin and amyloid[46] may be present in some tumours. Many basal cell epitheliomas are associated with a dermal chronic inflammatory cell host response.

The superficial type of basal cell epithelioma consists of lobules and islands of tumour 'budding-off' from several adjacent areas of epidermis. This variety of lesion rarely exhibits deep invasion, tending to grow in a horizontal fashion over long periods of time.

The morphoeic or sclerosing form of tumour consists of thin strands of basaloid cells embedded in a distinctive fibrous stroma (Figure 1.16). These tumours may be deeply invasive and their borders may be difficult to define histologically.

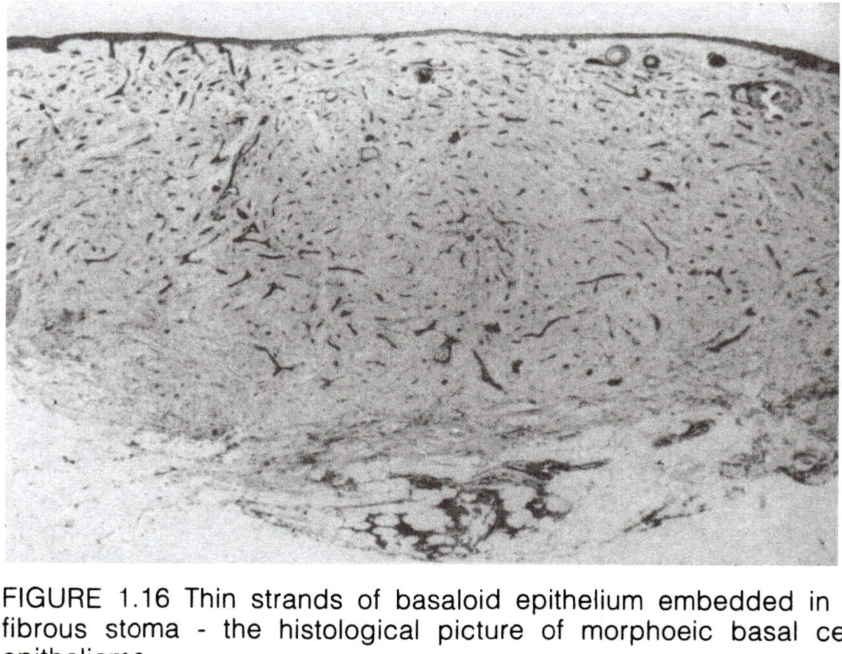

FIGURE 1.16 Thin strands of basaloid epithelium embedded in a fibrous stoma - the histological picture of morphoeic basal cell epithelioma

Squamous cell carcinoma

This tumour is less common than basal cell epithelioma (comparative incidences vary from 1:2 to 1:6, squamous cell epithelioma to basal cell carcinoma in various series) but has a capacity to metastasize. Sites that have a reputation for early lymph node metastasis include the genital area and the lips. The aetiological factors important in the development of squamous cell carcinoma are broadly similar to those relating to basal cell epithelioma, including exposure to ultraviolet light and other forms of radiation, genetic factors, chemical carcinogens and local (especially scarring) skin disease such as lupus vulgaris, lupus erythematosus[47] and dystrophic epidermolysis bullosa. The relationship of squamous cell carcinoma to Bowen's disease and actinic keratoses has been mentioned previously. In recent years, there has been considerable interest in the possible role of human papillomaviruses and other viruses in the histogenesis of at least some varieties of squamous cell carcinoma.

Clinical features (Figure 1.17)

Like basal cell epithelioma, this tumour most commonly occurs on exposed and sun-damaged skin such as the face or back of the hands, and may present as a hyperkeratotic crusted nodule or as an ulcer with a firm, indurated base. Lesions may develop from Bowen's disease and actinic keratoses and on occasions it may be difficult to distinguish clinically between a large proliferating actinic keratosis and an early basal cell epithelioma. A particular variety of squamous cell carcinoma known as carcinoma cuniculatum[48] occurs on the sole of the foot (Figure 1.18). Although it is rare, this tumour is often initially diagnosed as a viral wart and grows in a relentless locally destructive way. Histology reveals a very well-differentiated proliferation of squamous epithelium and this may also lead to a wrong diagnosis. A viral aetiology has been suggested for carcinoma cuniculatum and surgery is the treatment of choice for this lesion.

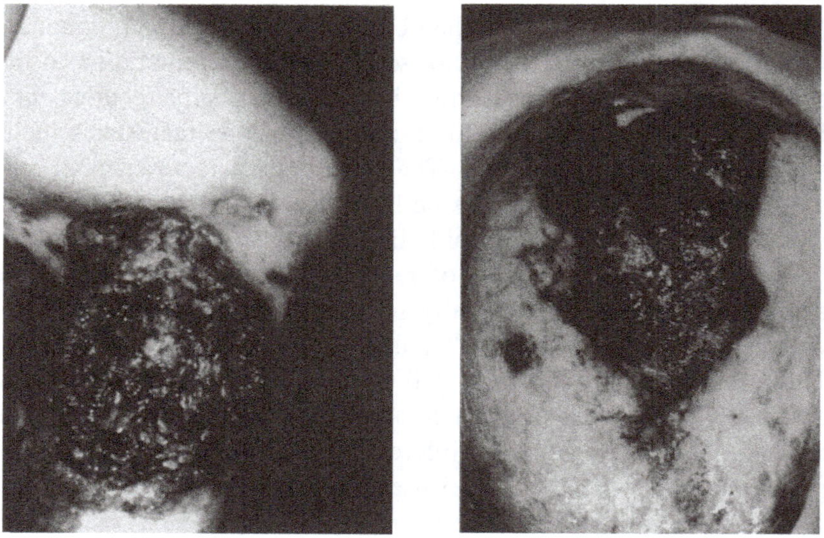

FIGURE 1.17 Two examples of squamous cell carcinoma arising (left) in a burn scar on the leg and (right) on scalp skin previously treated by radiotherapy for tinea capitis

Histology[49]

The histological appearance of squamous cell carcinoma varies considerably, depending on the degree of differentiation of the tumour. Most lesions show an irregular proliferation of squamous epithelium arising from either the epidermis or adnexal structures. Mitotic figures and varying degrees of keratinocyte cytological and nuclear atypia are seen. Acantholysis is common in carcinomas arising in actinic keratoses. Most lesions show, at least in some areas, a degree of squamous differentiation and small foci of keratinization; however, some anaplastic tumours may be completely undifferentiated, spindle cell variants often being difficult to separate from soft tissue sarcomas and spindle cell melanoma. In these circumstances the use of monoclonal antibodies and other markers (such as antibodies to keratin, epithelial membrane antigen and S100 protein) may help in achieving a correct diagnosis. In common with most pre-malignant and malignant conditions of the skin, a chronic inflammatory cell infiltrate of lymphocytes and plasma cells is often present at the deep margins of squamous cell epithelioma. The often difficult histological distinction of squamous cell epithelioma from keratoacanthoma has already been discussed.

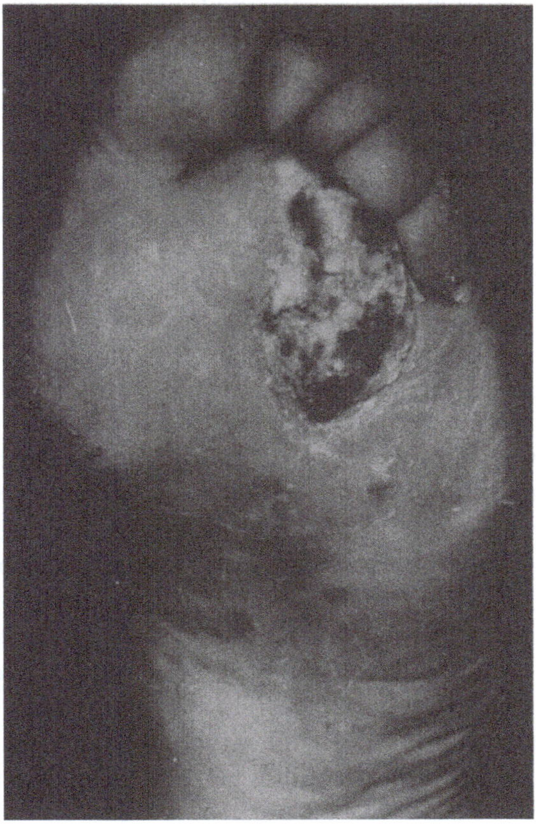

FIGURE 1.18 Carcinoma cuniculatum affecting the sole of the foot. This lesion was originally mis-diagnosed as a viral wart

Management of basal cell epithelioma and squamous cell carcinoma

The management of cutaneous cancer involves tumour prevention, the treatment of pre-cancer, the clinical and histological diagnosis of individual lesions, the correct choice and use of treatment modalities and appropriate follow-up. Education of the public, particularly regarding avoidance of over-exposure to sunlight and other forms of irradiation, is extremely important and programmes to disseminate information about the causes of skin cancer and how to avoid it are already reaping benefits in many countries. The correct diagnosis of tumours is an obvious prerequisite for the correct choice of treatment and aspects of clinical and histological diagnosis have already been considered. There are nowadays many effective modalities available for the treatment of basal cell epithelioma and squamous cell carcinoma of the skin, and a full discussion of the relative merits of different therapies is beyond the scope of this chapter. Readers are referred to the excellent review by Albright[50].

A multidisciplinary approach to management of skin cancer is the ideal, with the patient being seen by a dermatologist, surgeon and radiotherapist/oncologist in a combined tumour clinic. The choice of treatment depends on various factors, the most important of which concern the lesion itself, the patient and the resources available at the hospital or treatment centre. Factors relating to the lesion include size and site, histology, the presence or absence of metastases, whether the tumour is primary or recurrent, and the history and nature of any previous treatment. Patient-related factors include age and general health, the distance a patient lives from the treatment centre, and the patient's personal preference. As many cutaneous cancers can be treated equally well by surgical techniques as by radiotherapy (and very occasionally by chemotherapy), the choice of treatment method will also depend on the expertise and experience of the clinician as well as the facilities and equipment available.

Surgery

There are now a wealth of surgical techniques that have been used with great success in the management of skin cancer. These include excision with simple closure or plastic reconstruction, electrosurgery, curettage and cautery, Moh's micrographic surgery, cryotherapy and various laser techniques. Simple excision is an important and appropriate modality for many small basal and squamous cell tumours and curettage and cautery[51] and cryotherapy techniques are particularly useful for multiple tumours. Moh's micrographic surgery (originally chemosurgery), although time-consuming and not practical and economical for treating small and uncomplicated lesions, has proved itself of great value in the management of large and recurrent tumours, particularly when these occur adjacent to important vital structures. The advantages of surgery over radiotherapy include the availability of the whole specimen for histological evaluation and the fact that the treatment is often completed in one operation. Surgery may be preferred to radiotherapy for pigmented and ulcerated lesions, where the extent of the tumour is ill-defined, and for recurrences after radiotherapy.

Radiotherapy

Just as there is a wide range of surgical techniques available for the management of cutaneous carcinomas, several different forms of radiotherapy are also available. Orthovoltage radiotherapy is suitable for many tumours. A typical treatment regime for a basal cell epithelioma, for instance, might be 4000 cGy at 90V fractionated in 6–8 treatments over about 4–6 weeks. Electron-beam[52] therapy has a particular advantage when treating basal or squamous cell tumours overlying bone or cartilage. It is highly desirable before radiotherapy of any malignant skin lesion to carry out a biopsy for histological confirmation of the clinical diagnosis. Radiotherapy is a non-invasive procedure, which makes it suitable for unfit patients for whom surgery would require a general anaesthetic. Cosmetic results may also be superior to those of surgery when treating certain tumours, particularly where surgery would necessitate skin grafting. Radiotherapy also has a role in the palliation of widespread or inoperable disease.

Other treatment modalities

Systemic chemotherapy is rarely of importance in the management of primary (stage 1) cutaneous carcinoma, but may be extremely useful in the treatment of metastatic disease. Topical chemotherapy with 5-fluorouracil ointment for actinic keratoses and Bowen's disease has already been mentioned, as has the role of etretinate in the prophylaxis of epithelial cancer.

The proper approach to the management of cutaneous cancer involves education, prevention and a flexible approach to the choice of treatment. The many advances in therapeutic techniques developed in the last decade, together with the fact that many more patients are presenting to their physician with early lesions, has made skin cancer one of the most curable malignant diseases of man.

ACKNOWLEDGEMENTS

I am most grateful to Mrs Denise Venables for her expert secretarial assistance. The author is in receipt of a grant from the Dunhill Trust.

References

1. Greene, M.H., Clark, W.H. and Tucker, M.A. *et al.* (1985). Acquired precursors of cutaneous malignant melanoma. The familial dysplastic nevus syndrome. *New Engl. J. Med.*, **312**, 91–7
2. Rasmussen, J.E. (1975). A syndrome of trichoepitheliomas, milia and cylindromas. *Arch. Dermatol.*, **111**, 610–14
3. Kraemer, K.H., Lee, M.M. and Scotto, J. (1987). Xeroderma pigmentosum. *Arch. Dermatol.*, **123**, 241–50
4. Gorlin, R.J. (1987). Nevoid basal-cell carcinoma syndrome. *Medicine*, **66**, 98–113
5. Sorahan, T. and Grimley, R.P. (1985). The aetiological significance of sunlight and fluorescent lighting in malignant melanoma: A case-control study. *Br. J. Cancer*, **52**, 765–9
6. Fergin, P.E., Chu, A.C. and MacDonald, D.M. (1981). Basal cell carcinoma complicating naevus sebaceus. *Clin. Exp. Dermatol.*, **6**, 111–5
7. Altman, J. and Mehregan, A.H. (1971). Inflammatory linear verrucose epidermal naevus. *Arch. Dermatol.*, **104**, 385–9
8. Kaidbey, K.H. and Kurban, A.K. (1971). Dermatitic epidermal naevus. *Arch. Dermatol.*, **104**, 166–71

9. Solomon, L.M., Fretzin, D.F. and Dewald, R.L. (1968). The epidermal nevus syndrome. *Arch. Dermatol.*, **97**, 273–85
10. Demetree, J.W., Lang, P.G. and St. Clair, J.T. (1979). Unilateral, linear, zosteriform epidermal nevus with acantholytic dyskeratosis. *Arch. Dermatol.*, **115**, 875–7
11. Su, W.P.D. (1982). Histopathologic varieties of epidermal nevus. A study of 160 cases. *Am. J. Dermatopathol.*, **4**, 161–70
12. Breuninger, H. and Schippert, W. (1984). Combined application of dermatome and high-speed fraise in treatment of an extensive epidermal verrucous nevus. *Z. Hautkr.*, **60**, 356–63
13. Abdel-Aal, M.A.M. (1983). Treatment of systematized verrucous epidermal naevus by aromatic retinoid (Ro. 10–9359). *Clin. Exp. Dermatol,*, **8**, 647–50
14. Berman, A. and Winkelmann, R.K. (1982). Seborrheic keratoses. Appearance in course of exfoliative erythroderma and regression associated with histologic mononuclear cell inflammation. *Arch. Dermatol.*, **118**, 615–18
15. Holdiness, M.R. (1986). The sign of Leser-Trélat. *Int. J. Dermatol.*, **25**, 564–72
16. Braun-Falco, O. and Weissmann, I. (1978). Stukkokeratosen. Ubersicht und eigene Beobachtungen. *Hautarzt*, **29**, 573–7
17. Hairston, M.A., Reed, R.J. and Derbes, V.J. (1964). Dermatosis papulosa nigra. *Arch. Dermatol.*, **89**, 655–8
18. Wilson Jones, E. and Wells, G.C. (1966). Degos' acanthoma (acanthome à cellules claires). *Arch. Dermatol.*, **94**, 286–94
19. Trau, H., Fisher, B.K. and Schewach-Millet, M. (1980). Multiple clear cell acanthomas. *Arch. Dermatol.*, **116**, 433–4
20. Rook, A. and Whimster, I. (1979). Keratoacanthoma - a thirty year retrospect. *Br. J. Dermatol.*, **100**, 41–7
21. Stoll, D.M. and Ackerman, A.B. (1980). Subungual keratoacanthoma. *Am. J. Dermatopathol.*, **2**, 265–71
22. Janecka, I.P., Wolff, M., Crikelair, G.F. and Cosman, B. (1978). Aggressive histological features of keratoacanthoma. *J. Cutaneous Pathol.*, **4**, 342–8
23. Piscioli, F., Zumiani, G., Boi, S. and Cristofolini, M. (1984). A gigantic, metastasizing keratoacanthoma. *Am. J. Dermatopathol.*, **6**, 123–9
24. Weedon, D. and Barnett, L. (1975). Keratoacanthoma centrifugum marginatum. *Arch. Dermatol.*, **111**, 1024–6
25. Winkelmann, R.K. and Brown, J. (1968). Generalized eruptive keratoacanthoma. *Arch. Dermatol.*, **97**, 615–23
26. Ferguson-Smith, M.A., Wallace, D.C., James, Z.H. and Renwick, J.H. (1971). Multiple self-healing squamous epithelioma. *Birth Defects: Original Article Series*, **7**, 157–63
27. Shaw, J.C. and White, C.R. (1986). Treatment of multiple keratoacanthomas with oral isotretinoin. *J. Am. Acad. Dermatol.*, **15**, 1079–82
28. Cristofolini, M., Piscioli, F., Zumiani, G. and Scappini, P. (1985). The role of etretinate (Tegison; Tigason) in the management of keratoacanthoma. *J. Am. Acad. Dermatol.*, **12**, 633–8
29. Sayama, S. and Tagami, H. (1983). Treatment of keratoacanthoma with intralesional bleomycin. *Br. J. Dermatol.*, **109**, 449–52
30. Goette, D.K. (1983). Treatment of keratoacanthoma with topical fluorouracil. *Arch. Dermatol.*, **119**, 951–3
31. Eubanks, S.W., Gentry, R.H., Patterson, J.W. and May, D.L. (1982). Treatment

of multiple keratoacanthomas with intralesional fluorouracil. *J. Am. Acad. Dermatol.*, **7,** 126–9

32. Marks, R. (1987). Nonmelanotic skin cancer and solar keratoses. The quiet 20th century epidemic. *Int. J. Dermatol.*, **26,** 201–5
33. Wolff, H.H. and Lincke-Plewig, H. (1982). Lichenoide keratose. *Hautarzt,* **33,** 651–3
34. Subrt, P., Jorizzo, J.L., Apisarnthanarax, P., Head, E.S. and Smith, E.B. (1983). Spreading pigmented actinic keratosis. *J. Am. Acad. Dermatol.*, **8,** 63–7
35. Wade, T.R. and Ackerman, A.B. (1978). The many faces of solar keratoses. *J. Dermatol. Surg. Oncol.*, **4,** 730–4
36. Rahbari, H. and Pinkus, H. (1978). Large cell acanthoma. One of the actinic keratoses. *Arch. Dermatol.*, **114,** 49–52
37. Ackerman, A.B. and Reed, R.J. (1973). Epidermolytic variant of solar keratosis. *Arch. Dermatol.*, **107,** 104–6
38. Moriarty, M., Dunn, J., Darrach, A., Lambe, R. and Brick, I. (1982). Etretinate in treatment of actinic keratosis. A double-blind crossover study. *Lancet,* **1,** 364–5
39. Kao, G.F. (1986). Carcinoma arising in Bowen's Disease. *Arch. Dermatol.*, **122,** 1124–6
40. Miki, Y., Kawatsu, T., Matsuda, K., Machino, H. and Kubo, K. (1982). Cutaneous and pulmonary cancers associated with Bowen's Disease. *J. Am. Acad. Dermatol.*, **6,** 26–31
41. Scarborough, D.A., Bisaccia, E.P. and Yoder, F.W. (1982). Solitary pigmented Bowen's Disease. *Arch. Dermatol.*, **118,** 954–5
42. Kimura, S. (1982). Bowenoid papulosis of the genitalia. *Int. J. Dermatol.*, **21,** 432–6
43. Rustin, M.H.A., Chambers, T.J. and Munro, D.D. (1984). Post-traumatic basal cell carcinomas. *Clin. Exp. Dermatol.*, **9,** 379–83
44. Pollack, S.V., Goslen, J.B., Sherertz, E.F. and Jegasothy, B.V. (1982). The biology of basal cell carcinoma: A review. *J. Am. Acad. Dermatol.*, **7,** 569–77
45. Domarus, H.V. and Stevens, P.J. (1984). Metastatic basal cell carcinoma. *J. Am. Acad. Dermatol.*, **10,** 1043–60
46. Looi, L.M. (1983). Localized amyloidosis in basal cell carcinoma. A pathological study. *Cancer,* **52,** 1833–6
47. Millard, L.G. and Barker, D.J. (1978). Development of squamous cell carcinoma in chronic discoid lupus erythematosus. *Clin. Exp. Dermatol.*, **3,** 161–6
48. McKee, P.H., Wilkinson, J.D., Black, M.M. and Whimster, I.W. (1981). Carcinoma (epithelioma) cuniculatum: a clinico-pathological study of nineteen cases and review of the literature. *Histopathology,* **5,** 425–36
49. Wade, T.R. and Ackerman, A.B. (1978). The many faces of squamous-cell carcinomas. *J. Dermatol. Surg. Oncol.*, **4,** 291–4
50. Albright, S.D. (1982). Treatment of skin cancer using multiple modalities. *J. Am. Acad. Dermatol.*, **7,** 143–71
51. Spiller, W.F. and Spiller, R.F. (1984). Treatment of basal cell epithelioma by curettage and electrodesiccation. *J. Am. Acad. Dermatol.*, **11,** 808–14
52. Miller, R.A. and Spittle, M.F. (1982). Electron beam therapy for difficult cutaneous basal and squamous cell carcinoma. *Br. J. Dermatol.*, **106,** 429–36

2

THE DIAGNOSIS AND MANAGEMENT OF MALIGNANT MELANOMA

N.C. DAVIS

HISTORICAL ASPECTS

The first published account of a patient with melanoma – a secondary deposit with no known primary – was reported by John Hunter in 1787, although Hunter never described the disease as such. The original specimen is preserved in the Hunterian Museum of the Royal College of Surgeons of England. In 1820, William Norris, of Stourbridge, England, described the first case of melanoma in the English literature[1]. It was of a patient who died of disseminated melanoma. Norris was a pioneer in the understanding of melanoma[2]. Among other things, he was the first to report local recurrence following minimal excision; the first to advocate wide excision of the tumour and surrounding tissues; the first to note that neither medical nor surgical treatment was effective when the disease was widely disseminated; and the first to record melanoma in a family. Sir Jonathan Hutchinson described subungual melanoma in 1857 and later illustrated in 1892 and 1894 a series of cases, to which the title "Hutchinson's Melanotic Freckle" was applied. Sampson Handley, in 1907, advocated wide local excision and regional node dissection on the basis of an autopsy of a single patient with a very advanced melanoma. Such was his authority that this recommendation formed the basis of orthodox melanoma treatment for the ensuing fifty or more years. It is only in recent times that this policy of wide excision and routine node dissection has been questioned.

In the last twenty years, McGovern, Clark, Breslow and Ackerman have contributed greatly to the understanding of the pathology and biology of this fascinating tumour and have thereby significantly influenced its treatment.

EPIDEMIOLOGY[3]

The incidence of cutaneous malignant melanoma is rising in every Western country in which it has been studied. Queensland, occupying the northeast corner of Australia, has the highest incidence of melanoma in the world – 40 new cases per 100 000 of population in 1979–80. The crude incidence in the state has more than doubled since 1966. In contrast, the incidence in west of Scotland is only about 5 per 100 000.

Melanoma is largely a problem of white people. The great majority of cases arise in the skin of white caucasians. Any racial type of skin pigmentation seems to be protective. In Blacks and Orientals, the disease is less common and tends to occur in the less-pigmented areas such as the sole of the foot, the subungual region, the nasal or oral cavity, the anal canal and the vulva.

The aetiology is multifactorial. Genetic factors are said to be responsible for 11% of cases. Those of Celtic ancestry seem to be genetically predisposed to melanoma. These individuals often have fair complexions, red hair and a tendency to sunburn and freckle.

Apart from the constitutional make-up of the host, lifestyle and environmental exposure to sunlight are very important in the aetiology of melanoma.

There is a strong positive association between the degree of exposure to ultraviolet and the incidence of melanoma. In contrast with non-melanoma skin cancers, which appear to be influenced more by cumulative lifetime exposure to ultraviolet light, it may well be that sporadic instances of intense exposure to sun are more likely to induce melanoma than simple duration of exposure.

Certainly, episodes of severe sunburn, especially in childhood and adolescence, are often noted in the past history of patients with melanoma. It is interesting that studies of migrants who arrived in Australia after the age of nineteen years have a relatively low incidence of melanoma in spite of many subsequent years in the country. The geographic distribution of melanoma correlates negatively with latitude on a world scale. The closer one is to the equator, the more likely one is to develop a melanoma if one has white skin.

Outdoor workers have an excess incidence of melanomas on exposed sites of the body, yet, overall, the highest incidence and mortality rates occur in professional and managerial occupations, in persons of high socioeconomic status and in those with indoor as against outdoor occupations.

Evidence is accumulating that occupational exposures to chemicals and to radiation may be important. A suggestion has been made, but not yet confirmed, that office work under fluorescent lighting is associated with an increased risk of melanoma. In considering occupational exposure, it should be remembered that, for financial reasons, fewer individuals in developed countries are now required to work outdoors. In contrast, exposure to sunlight by choice has increased. Many people from cold climates have vacations in sunny regions by the sea; lighter clothing is worn and more skin is exposed.

There is a statistical association between melanoma and a past history of skin cancer. Squamous and basal cell carcinomas are unequivocally associated with prolonged exposure to sunlight. They are very common in elderly people, especially those who work outdoors. One type of melanoma, that developing in a Hutchinson's melanotic freckle, appears to have a similar origin. These melanomas occur especially on the face of elderly people, and the surrounding skin shows evidence of sun damage.

About 50% of melanomas develop in a pre-existing naevus. There is a statistical correlation between the number of naevi present on an individual and the risk of developing a melanoma.

There now seems to be very little difference in the sex incidence but there is a significant difference in the site distribution in men and women. The commonest site in men is on the back of the trunk and in women on the lower limbs. Women in general, have a better prognosis than men.

Melanoma is exceedingly rare before puberty and its incidence increases with age. It is most common between 30 and 50 years of age – the most productive period of life.

There is a tendency for melanomas to run in families. Familial patients tend to be younger, of Celtic origin, and prone to develop multiple primary melanomas. Attention has been drawn recently to the dysplastic naevus syndrome, which may be either familial or sporadic (see later). Those suffering from this syndrome are more likely to develop multiple primaries than the population at large. However, familial dysplastic naevi are not common enough to make a major contribution to the total incidence of melanoma.

There is no overall relation between the prior use of oral contraceptives and the subsequent development of melanoma. Pregnancy neither increases risk of melanoma nor affects prognosis. Smokers have no higher incidence, but are more likely to develop metastatic melanoma and have a worse prognosis. Patients after renal transplantation are likely to develop skin tumours, including melanoma. This is thought to be due to immunosuppressant drugs. There is no proven relationship between trauma and melanoma. This was originally suggested because of the frequent occurrence of melanoma on the sole of the foot in the barefoot Black African. But melanoma occurs also on the sole of the foot of Black Americans, who regularly wear shoes.

Frequent washing – very common in Europeans living in hot climates – has been suggested as causing melanoma by removing the protective skin secretions.

Melanoma is one of the few malignant tumours that has been demonstrated to exhibit spontaneous regression. This has prompted close study of the immunology of the disease.

CLINICAL PRESENTATION

Melanoma is a potentially lethal disease that can be diagnosed clinically in the majority of cases without any sophisticated techniques. All one needs to do is listen to the patient when he or she tells you about the mole, and then examine the tumour carefully in a good light, preferably with a magnifying lens. Our experience has shown that any competent medical practitioner can be taught to recognize a melanoma on the basis of a history of some unusual change in a mole, and the appearance of irregularity in some aspect of the tumour. Naturally, the diagnosis has to be confirmed microscopically, but my point is that it should be rare for the clinician to be surprised when a pathologist reports a lesion as a malignant melanoma. One's whole effort should be towards diagnosing melanoma at the earliest biological stage, that is, when it is less than 0.76 mm thick or invading to Clark's levels I or II. This is now possible in over 50% of patients with melanoma in Queensland[4]. Patients with such early lesions are eminently curable[5].

CLINICAL DIAGNOSIS

A history of change in a pre-existing mole, or the continued growth of a new mole in an adult, is suggestive of malignancy . The most significant change is that which occurs over a period of weeks or months rather than over a few days. The latter change is rarely due to malignancy but is more commonly the result of infection (e.g., of an epidermal cyst underlying a benign naevus) or of trauma. It should be realized that some patients report that they have never noticed any change at all, even though the pigmented lesion is obviously different from any other mole present.

The development of malignancy in a mole should be suspected if any of the following occur.

1. Change in size. A pigmented lesion spreads out to cover a larger surface area.
2. Change in outline. The edge of the lesion, perhaps previously round, becomes indented or notched or otherwise irregular.
3. Change in colour. The usual change is for an ordinary brown mole to become darker or black, either uniformly or in part. Very characteristic is an irregularity of colour within the tumour itself, producing all shades or brown, blue, grey, red, black and pink. Depressed pale areas of depigmentation within the pigmented tumour are almost pathognomonic of malignant melanoma and will be seen microscopically to be areas of local tumour regression. Sometimes, a mole develops a pink or amelanotic tumour that, to an inexperienced observer, may resemble a granuloma or

an infected lesion. An intensity of pigmentation at the periphery of a mole is suspicious.

4. Change in elevation. A previously flat lesion becomes thickened and readily palpable with the finger tip. Alternatively, one or more nodules, pigmented or otherwise, develop within the tumour.
5. Change in the surface characteristics. The earliest change may be a loss of normal skin markings. A smooth mole may become rough, scaly or ulcerated.
6. Change in the surrounding tissues. Lumps, either pigmented or non-pigmented, developing in the immediate vicinity of a mole may possibly be satellite tumours.
7. Development of symptoms and signs. One of the most characteristic symptoms, suggestive of malignancy, is a tingling, an intermittent itchiness or a sense of awareness of the presence of a mole. Serous discharge requiring a dressing or recurrent minor bleeding after trivial trauma is highly suspicious.

CLINICO-PATHOLOGICAL TYPES OF MELANOMA[7]

There are four common clinico-pathological types of melanoma. The experienced observer can diagnose these types by their appearance, but it is sufficient for most practitioners to recognize that the lesion is a melanoma.

1. *Superficial spreading melanoma* (Figure 2.1). This is the most common (64%) in our series. It may occur on any part of the body and is usually greater than 0.5 cm in diameter. A variegated pattern of colour and an irregular edge is characteristic. The lesion is usually palpable and nodule(s) may develop within the tumour. These may be blue, black or pink. It is possible to diagnose this type of melanoma when the tumour cells are confined to the epidermis, i.e. when it is a melanoma *in situ*. Such lesions are flat, often with irregular scalloped margins, are somewhat symmetrical, irregular in their pigmentation, and are usually greater

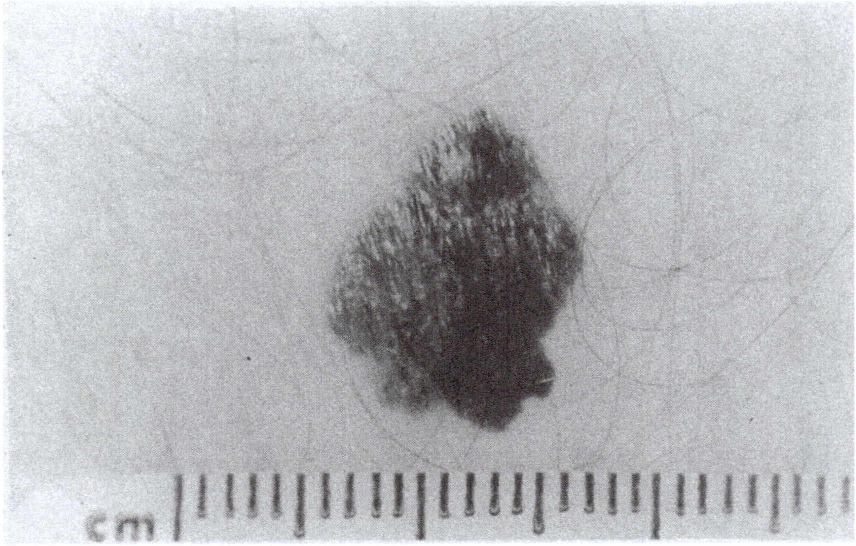

FIGURE 2.1 Superficial spreading melanoma

than 5 mm in diameter. We do not like euphemistic terms such as active junction naevus, atypical melanocytic hyperplasia or premalignant melanoma used for a melanoma *in situ*.

2. *Nodular melanoma.* (Figure 2.2). Nodular melanoma is less common (28%), but more malignant. It may occur on any part of the body. There is no antecedent spreading of pigmentation. When first noted clinically, this lesion is always palpable and usually convex in shape. The colour, in contrast with other melanomas, is commonly uniform and is usually blue, grey or black. It may be pink or amelanotic. However, close inspection will commonly show some pigmentation at the base of the lesion. It is sharply delineated from the surrounding tissue, has a smooth surface and a regular outline. Ulceration may occur early in the disease, leading to weeping or bleeding. This is the most difficult type of melanoma to diagnose.

3. *Lentigo maligna melanoma.* (Syn. melanoma arising in a Hutchinson's melanotic freckle) (Figure 2.3). This is less common (7%) and least malignant. It occurs most frequently on the

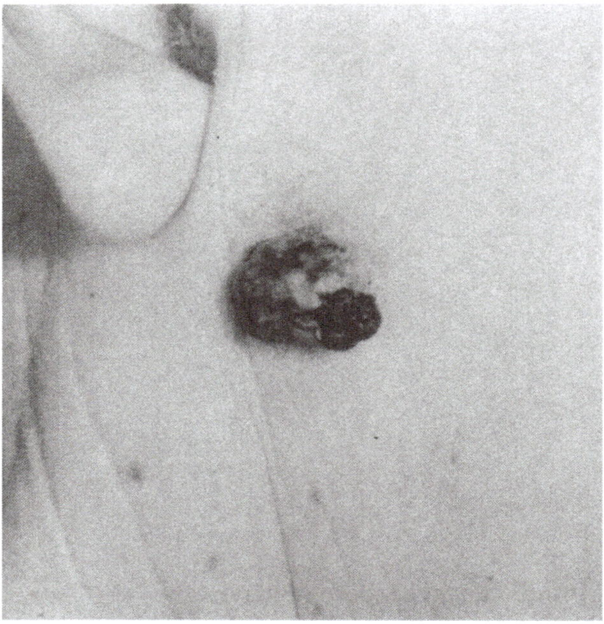

FIGURE 2.2 Nodular melanoma

face of persons over 60 years. It may occur on any part of the body habitually exposed to the sun. It begins as an irregularly pigmented, flat, brown macule which grows very slowly over a period of 10–15 years, advancing and regressing in various areas. There is a great variation in colour from brown to tan to black within the tumour itself. Malignant change is recognized by thickening and the development of discrete tumour nodules. It may ultimately grow to a diameter of 4–6 cm. A very irregular outline is characteristic.

4. *Acral-lentiginous melanoma.* (Figure 2.4) This is the least common type (1%), and may have a poor prognosis because of delayed diagnosis. It characteristically occurs on the soles, especially in coloured people, such as Negroes and Orientals. Whereas it constitutes only a tiny proportion of melanoma in white Caucasians, it has been reported as high as 40% in Japanese and even higher in Africans. Even though the lesion may be large (3 cm or more in diameter) it is often disregarded because of

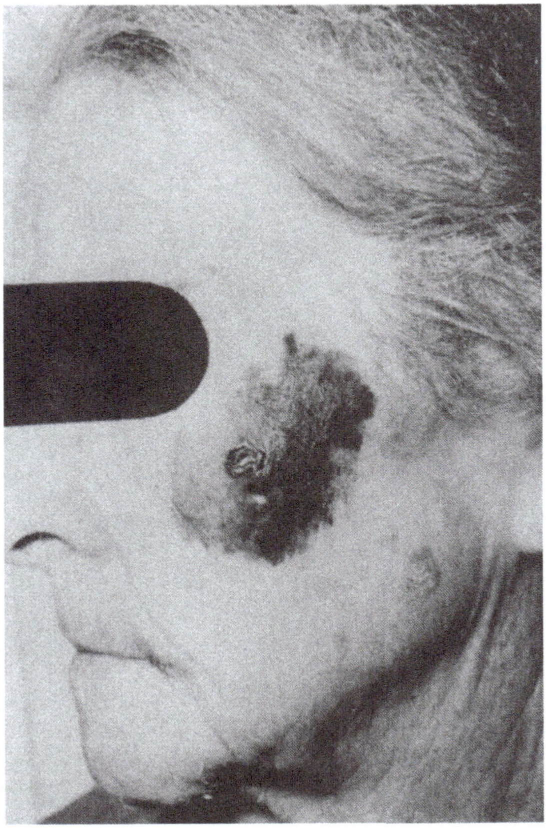

FIGURE 2.3 Lentigo maligna melanoma

its anatomical situation, and is thought to be a minor infection, a blood blister or a plantar wart. It often starts as a brown-black stain, apparently in the skin itself, but later becomes raised, ulcerated and fungating.

Acral-lentiginous melanomas may also occur on the palms of the hands, in the mucosae and beneath the nail-bed. Subungual melanomas tend to involve the thumb and the great toe. They often start as a brown/black streak under the nail. As the lesion grows, it destroys the nail, which is replaced by a raw granulating surface. It is commonly mistaken for a subungual haematoma or whitlow. Usually, there is enough pigment in the lesion or at the periphery to make the diagnosis.

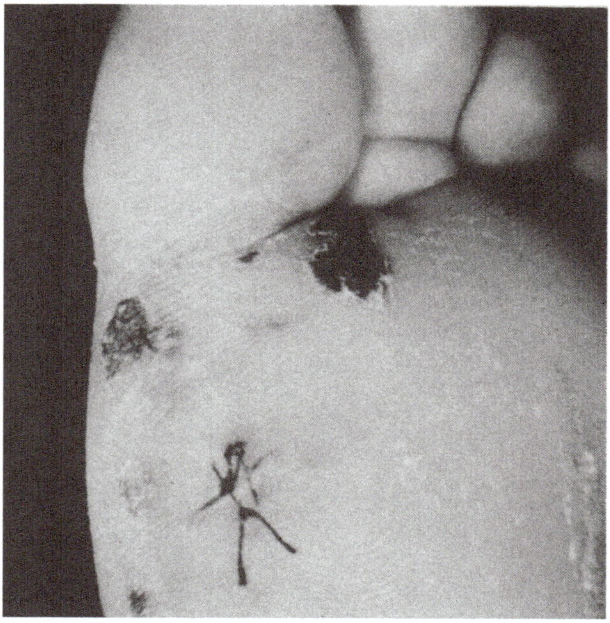

FIGURE 2.4 Acral-lentiginous melanoma

An uncommon but important type of melanoma is the desmoplastic melanoma. It tends to occur on the face or neck and is difficult to recognize unless there is some overlying pigmentation. A characteristic feature is induration that may suggest a fibroma or fibrosarcoma. The tumour cells in this type of melanoma infiltrate deeply, often beyond the clinically recognizable extent of the tumour. For this reason, they have a great tendency to recur locally after excision and they frequently give rise to distant metastases.

Patients sometimes present for the first time with metastatic melanoma. This may take the form of small pigmented or non-pigmented satellites in the region of the primary tumour, or subcutaneous lumps in the vicinity or elsewhere on the body.

Some patients present with secondary melanoma in the regional lymph nodes and no known primary tumour. Lymph nodes clinically involved with tumour have the following characteristics. They are palpable, usually greater than 1 cm in diameter and often round. Sometimes they develop very rapidly, with subcutaneous bruising.

In these circumstances, the secondary deposits may become smaller while under observation. The nodes are characteristically firm, rubbery and mobile. It is rare for them to be fixed to vital structures.

It is not uncommon for a patient to be operated on for a cerebral tumour and for it found to be a secondary melanoma.

It is important always to examine the patient with a primary melanoma carefully in case there are other primary melanomas present. Multiple primaries occur in about 4% of cases.

DIFFERENTIAL DIAGNOSIS[6]

Benign melanocytic tumours

No two lesions are so alike in appearance as moles and melanomas but so different in their subsequent behaviour. Unlike melanomas, benign moles typically exhibit a uniformity of colour, and a regularity or pattern and outline. Hairs often grow in benign moles but rarely do so in melanomas, except on the scalp. The clinician should learn to recognize the following types of benign naevi.

Junctional naevus

The junctional naevus is a smooth, flat, hairless mole. The colour is a uniform dark brown or black, although there may be dots of black pigment present. The normal skin markings are usually visible. The outline is well-defined and there are rarely any indentations. Its size varies from a few millimetres to a centimetre in diameter. It may occur anywhere on the body.

Naevi on the palms, soles, genitalia and mucous membranes are said to be junctional, but many are compound naevi. Junctional naevi occur any time after birth and they are common moles in children before puberty. Their great importance lies in the fact that they may develop into a malignant melanoma, although this is denied by some workers. They rarely become malignant before puberty. In fact, most junctional naevi remain benign throughout life and evolve with the passage of time into compound or intradermal naevi.

Compound naevus

Compound naevi are composed of junctional and intradermal elements. They are most common in adolescents. They are a brown/black mole usually less than 1 cm in size. The surface is elevated and nodular. There is commonly a brown macular ring around the periphery. They may be hairy and are often clinically indistinguishable from an intradermal naevus. By virtue of its raised centre, the compound naevus bears a superficial resemblance to a malignant melanoma. While it may develop into a malignant melanoma, it usually remains quite benign and matures into an intradermal naevus.

Intradermal naevus

Intradermal naevus is the common mature mole of adults. It may occur anywhere but is rare on the palms, soles and genitalia. It is most common on the scalp and face of adults. It varies in size from a few millimetres to several centimetres. It may be flat and smooth, raised and warty, pigmented or non-pigmented, and sessile or pedunculated. It often contains coarse hairs. It is quite benign and rarely becomes malignant.

Blue naevus

Blue naevus is a rather uncommon dark-blue or black hairless lesion, usually less than 0.5 cm in diameter. It is slightly elevated, indurated and easily palpable. The overlying epidermis is remarkably smooth and the outline is regular. It is most common on the head and neck, on the dorsum of hands and feet, and on the buttocks. It is rather more common in women than men and has usually shown little change since it was noticed initially. It is almost always benign.

Halo naevus

The halo naevus is a benign lesion occurring mainly on the backs of children and adolescents. There is a brown papular pigmented lesion in the centre of a well-circumscribed pale white circle of depigmented skin. With time, these lesions resolve, leaving a small white patch. The change is probably the result of some immunological process.

Spitz naevus (Syn. juvenile melanoma, compound melanocytoma)

Spitz naevus is a rapidly growing pigmented lesion occurring particularly in children but not uncommonly in adults. Usually, it is less than 1 cm in size, and pink or red, but occasionally it is brown or black. It may be soft or hard, usually dome-shaped but sometimes sessile or pedunculated. It may occur anywhere on the body. It can be difficult to recognize clinically. Its main importance is its histological resemblance to melanoma, and even experienced pathologists have difficulty in distinguishing the two. However, very few progress to become malignant.

Solar (senile) lentigo

Solar lentigo occurs as brown patches on sun-damaged skin, particularly on the backs of hands and wrists of elderly individuals. It can be distinguished from melanoma in that it is usually flat and much more uniform in colour, size and outline.

Dysplastic naevi

Dysplastic naevi are dealt with in a special section (see below).

Other benign skin lesions

Seborrhoeic keratosis (Syn. senile wart, acanthotic naevus, pigmented basal cell papilloma)

Seborrhoeic keratosis is a slowly growing raised lesion varying from a few millimetres to 2 cm or more in size. It develops singly or in large numbers on the trunk, face and neck of middle-aged people. It may be yellow, brown, grey or black. Some are dome-shaped or pedunculated with a smooth shiny surface, but close inspection will usually show pits or indentations filled with keratin. Some seborrhoeic keratoses are flat and sessile, with a rather warty or greasy surface while others are dry and rough. They sometimes seem as if they are merely stuck on the skin, and parts can easily be picked off it. Some pieces of the lesion may flake off with minor trauma, leading to slight bleeding and causing both the patient and his doctor to think it might be a melanoma.

Sclerosing angioma (dermatofibroma)

Sclerosing angioma occurs as a small indurated nodule feeling like lead shot in the skin. It is usually less than 1cm in diameter and is found especially on the legs in women. Most are pink, but some are pigmented – although the colour is blue rather than black. It is these that may closely resemble a malignant melanoma. The surface is smooth and hairless, and the outline is regular and well circumscribed. Its induration and adherence to the skin should allow it to be distinguished from a melanoma.

Pyogenic granuloma

Pyogenic granuloma often develops rapidly after a minor injury. It usually presents as a dull-red, pedunculated tumour. The surface may be ulcerated and crusted. Usually, it is compressible and this may be a distinctive feature. It has a tendency to bleed with minor trauma and this causes confusion with melanoma. It may closely resemble an amelanotic melanoma, but the latter usually has a trace of pigment at its base.

Haemangioma

Classically, a haemangioma is small, bluish-red in colour with a smooth raised surface and a well-defined edge. It can usually be diagnosed by compression with a glass slide, which produces a significant reduction in intensity of colour and of elevation. Thrombosis in a haemangioma produces an induration and blue/black colour very suggestive, in some cases, of melanoma.

Intracutaneous haemorrhage

Haemorrhage, following minor trauma, into the cornified layer of the epidermis or into the nail-bed can resemble a melanoma. It may occur on the heel of athletes and cause anxiety because of its black colour and irregular shape. Inspection with a magnifying lens will often show skin markings to be normal and that the colour is reddish blue rather than black.

MALIGNANT SKIN TUMOURS

Pigmented basal cell carcinoma

Basal cell carcinomas are very common in white Caucasians living in tropical and subtropical regions. They tend to occur in middle age, particularly on exposed surfaces such as the head and neck. Some are pigmented and these are often difficult to distinguish from melanomata. Most are less than 2 cm in size. They are bluish-black in colour and the pigment is unevenly distributed, occurring particularly towards the periphery. The edge is raised and smooth and slightly indurated. On stretching, they exhibit a dark, pearly appearance and some tiny venules may be visible. The surface is smooth but it may be nodular, cystic or ulcerated. In general, hairs are absent.

Pigmented squamous cell carcinoma

These are less commonly seen than the above and may present with a scaly surface, an indurated nodule or an ulcer. They may look suspicious if they have recently experienced trauma leading to bleeding.

DYSPLASTIC NAEVI[8]

Dysplastic naevi are acquired pigmented lesions of the skin whose clinical and histological definitions are still evolving. They were first recognized and described by Clark and associates in 1978 because of their unusual appearance and increased frequency in certain families who suffered from melanoma. Dysplastic naevi most commonly occur as multiple lesions in an individual, but they may be solitary.

Typical dysplastic naevi are 5–12 mm in diameter and tend to be larger than common naevi. They have both macular and papular components. The surface has been described as pebbly and their borders are often irregular and ill defined. The margins tend to be indistinct and to fade into adjacent normal skin. Their colour is variegated, ranging from tan to dark brown on a pink or erythematous background. Dysplastic naevi sometimes clinically resemble melanomas. Their distribution is often different from that of common naevi in that they tend to occur on covered areas, such as the trunk and scalp. In contrast with most young adults who may have up to 25 benign naevi, an individual with dysplastic naevi may have more than 100 lesions. They tend to appear in adolescence and new lesions may develop up to the age of 35 years. Dysplastic naevi can be inherited or may be sporadic. Familial dysplastic naevi can be inherited as an autosomal dominant trait. The presence of multiple dysplastic naevi in two or more family members has been termed the dysplastic naevus syndrome. The importance of the dysplastic naevus syndrome is that individuals with the condition are believed to have an increased risk of developing a malignant melanoma. The overall lifetime risk of this has been estimated at 10%. The prevalence of dysplastic naevi in the general population is thought to be about 5%. Dysplastic naevi are both markers of and precursors for familial melanoma. There is still much controversy about these lesions. Dixon and Ackerman[9] claim that dysplastic naevi are variants of compound and junctional naevi and that microscopically less than 5% of melanomas develop from dysplastic naevi. They believe that the majority of melanomas begin *de novo* and not from cells of melanocytic naevi of any kind.

The management of patients with the dysplastic naevus syndrome is still somewhat controversial. It is desirable to excise at least one naevus for microscopic examination, but the wholesale removal of all the naevi is undesirable. Certainly, any naevus that changes should be excised and examined. The patient should be warned of the possibility of developing melanomas. Some clinicians photograph the lesions to serve as a record. The patient should be examined every 3–6 months and advised to avoid excess exposure to sun. The first-degree relatives should also be examined to see whether they have the condition.

MICROSTAGING OF MELANOMA

Very valuable work has been done by pathologists in this area in the last twenty years. Clark *et al*[10] 1969 defined five microanatomical levels of invasion of the skin by tumour cells.

- Level I All tumour cells confined to the epidermis with no invasion through the basement membrane (melanoma in situ).
- Level II Tumour cells penetrating through the basement membrane into the papillary dermis but not extending into reticular dermis.
- Level III Tumour cells filling the papillary dermis and abutting against the reticular dermis but not invading it.
- Level IV Extension of tumour cells into the reticular dermis.
- Level V Tumour cells invading the subcutaneous fat.

There is a strong correlation between depth of invasion and prognosis. Survival decreases with increasing invasion. The problem with Clark's classification is that its application requires much experience on the part of the pathologist, particularly in estimating Level III[11]. A more accurate method of microstaging was developed by Breslow in 1970. He measured the thickness of the tumour with an ocular micrometer. The distances from the top of the granular layer or ulcer base to the deepest extension of the tumour is measured in millimetres, rounded up or down to the first figure beyond the decimal point.

Histological reporting

The pathologist has a vital role to play in guiding the clinician in the management of the patient with melanoma[12]. He should produce a full report containing the following information:

- Malignant melanoma - primary site
- Size of tumour in mm
- Histogenetic type
- Thickness to nearest 0.1 mm
- Clark's level (I-V)
- Ulceration - present/absent
- Mitotic rate/mm^2
- Local regression - present/absent
- Vascular or lymphatic invasion - present/absent
- Margins of excision in mm
- Tumour in excision margin - present/absent

Other features that are sometimes mentioned in special centres are the cross-sectional profiles, the cell type, the degree of melanogenesis, lymphocytic infiltration, solar degeneration, and whether there is an associated naevus either dysplastic or not.

If lymph nodes are removed, the pathologist should report the number of nodes present, the number involved by tumour, and the presence or absence of extracapsular invasion.

DECISIONS OF MANAGEMENT

When a patient consults his general practitioner about a mole, the doctor can reach only three conclusions about the diagnosis: it is innocent; it is malignant; or he does not know.

Benign lesions

Benign pigmented lesions typically exhibit an orderly array of colour, a regularity of pattern, a symmetry of outline, and a uniformity of surface, in contrast to melanomas. Coarse hair growing from a mole usually implies that it is innocent, but hairs may grow from melanomas on the scalp.
What innocent moles should be removed?

1. Moles undergoing any unusual change. This is because the clinical diagnosis might be wrong and the lesion might be malignant.
2. Naevi in areas subject to repeated trauma or irritation (because they are a constant annoyance).
3. Naevi that are flat and black or otherwise irregular, on the legs of women and backs of men, especially if greater than 0.5 cm in size (because of the high incidence of melanoma in these areas).
4. Moles on the soles of the feet, female genitalia, and mucosal surfaces (because of the poor prognosis if melanomas develop in these areas).
5. Moles in patients who are terrified of malignancy, perhaps because of family history of melanoma.
6. Children with solitary moles that are growing or attracting attention: they should have the mole removed before puberty. Melanoma is exceedingly rare before puberty and removal of such a mole before puberty is justifiable for prophylaxis.

If it is thought that a benign naevus should be removed, the mole should be totally excised with a minimal margin of skin. Some underlying fat may be removed but not the deep fascia. The operation is usually done under local anaesthesia and the specimen should always be sent for microscopic examination.

When in doubt

When the clinician is uncertain whether a particular mole is malignant or not, biopsy is usually indicated. Excisional biopsy is the method of choice. It should be done under local anaesthesia taking a small margin (e.g. 2 mm) of normal skin and fat only. The incision should be placed in the direction of the lymph drainage (and not necessarily in the direction of Langer's lines) so that any subsequent surgery is made easier. Incisional biopsy should generally be avoided except where the lesion is so large or anatomically so situated that complete removal cannot be performed simply. The area selected should include the thickest part of the lesion. Punch biopsy is similarly rarely indicated, but, if it is performed, the thickest part of the tumour should be taken. There is no indication for shave biopsy of a pigmented lesion and cautery to the base is potentially dangerous. The problem with incisional punch biopsy or shave biopsy is that not enough material may be provided to allow histological assessment of thickness, level, or morphological type, all of which influence subsequent management. While there is no evidence that a preliminary excision biopsy is harmful, the patient may be disadvantaged if the melanoma has been removed before he or she is seen by the surgeon. Patient may have become very distressed by the diagnosis, especially when it is unexpected. They may panic from an unjustified fear of early death or mutilating surgery. The incision may have been so placed as to make subsequent surgery unnecessarily mutilating. Clinical assessment of the regional nodes is made more difficult if the wound is inflamed, gaping, or has a haematoma.

In cases where the pathologist reports 'local excision is adequate', neither the patient nor his general practitioner may appreciate the need for further surgery. Incidentally, it is recommended that pathologists report that 'margins of excision are free of tumour' rather than 'excision is adequate', which is a value judgement. When the surgeon himself is in doubt about diagnosis, he may excise the lesion totally under local anaesthesia and await an urgent paraffin section, the report on which should be available within 48 hours. Tentative arrangements can be made to admit the patient to hospital for further surgery without delay. Alternatively, the surgeon may arrange for a frozen-section examination under general anaesthesia, if an experienced pathologist is available[13].

An experienced surgeon can often perform excisional biopsy on a suspicious lesion, taking sufficient margin of surrounding normal skin that this constitutes definitive treatment of the subsequently confirmed melanoma. This will avoid a second operation.

PROGNOSTIC FACTORS[14]

Sex

Numerous studies have shown that women have a better survival than men with melanoma.

Anatomical location

Patients with extremity melanomas have a better survival than those with their tumours on the trunk or head and neck. Lesions on scalp, vulva and sole of feet tend to do poorly. Day et al[15] reported a worse prognosis for patients with lesions on upper back, upper outer arm, neck and scalp (BANS), but this has not been confirmed.

Age

Patients over 45 years of age tend to present with thicker lesions and have a worse prognosis than younger patients.

Rate of growth

There is no doubt that some melanomas run a very rapid course. They are usually nodular melanomas, with a short history. They are deeply invasive, thick and ulcerated. Dissemination occurs soon after their appearance and medical treatment is of no avail.

Treatment at or prior to diagnosis

It is difficult to be sure what the effect is of inappropriate initial treatment of a melanoma. Certainly, diathermy or cautery to a melanoma is believed to lead to early dissemination and death.

Previous inadvertent cryotherapy to an unrecognized melanoma is often followed by a deeply invasive recurrence. Trauma does not convert a benign naevus into a melanoma, but repeated trauma to a melanoma cannot have a good effect, and may cause dissemination. Reference has been made above to incisional punch and shave biopsy. While there is no proof that they are actually harmful, they are inadvisable in most cases. In melanoma as in most cancers, it is the first definitive treatment that carries the greatest chance of cure.

Tumour thickness

The total vertical height of a melanoma is the single most important prognostic factor in stage I melanoma. Most other prognostic variables derive their predictive ability by a secondary correlation with tumour thickness. Numerous groups of thickness subsets have been measured for their prognostic value (e.g. less than 0.76 mm, 0.76–1.5 mm, greater than 1.5 mm), but the probability is that there are no 'natural breakpoints' and the relationship between thickness and mortality rate is a continuous event. Thickness is easier to measure and is more reproducible than the level of invasion. It should be remembered that some thin melanomas, especially those showing signs of local regression, metastasize and may cause death[16].

Level of invasion

There is an inverse correlation between increasing (Clark's) levels of invasion and survival. It should be noted that there is some variability of tumour thickness within each level of invasion and that the thickness correlates with survival better than does the level.

Ulceration

About 20% of melanomas may show microscopic evidence of ulceration. This feature is more common in thick melanomas, and in men. It is an independent prognostic variable and carries a poor prognosis.

Growth pattern

Ackerman has argued vigorously for a unifying concept of malignant melanoma[17]. He claims that all melanomas evolve in a similar way: all at first spread horizontally (superficially) within the epidermis and all may eventually extend vertically into the dermis. He states that the usually accepted classification into superficial spreading, nodular, lentigo maligna and acral lentiginous melanoma is unnecessary. None the less, it is conventional wisdom that patients with lentigo maligna melanoma do better than those with superficial spreading melanoma. These two types are associated with a better survival than nodular and acral lentiginous melanomas. If the maximum thickness of the tumour is correlated in any of those types of melanoma, the prognosis is roughly similar.

Pigmentation

Amelanotic melanomas are uncommon but have a worse prognosis. They are considerably thicker than highly pigmented tumours and are often diagnosed late.

Local regression

Regression seen in a primary melanoma does not imply that the host resistance is high and that there will be a good prognosis. In fact, those patients who present with secondary deposits and no known primary lesion presumably developed their metastases from a primary melanoma that underwent total regression.

Clinico-pathological stage

The presence of involved regional lymph nodes, satellite tumours, in-transit metastases and distant metastases all are associated with a poor prognosis.

Pregnancy

As stated above pregnancy does not affect the prognosis except in so far that it may cause delay in the institution of effective treatment.

Prognostic index

A prognostic index has been suggested by Schmoeckel and Braun-Falco[18]. It is defined as the product of the tumour thickness and the mitotic rate. Indices are reported as low, medium and high, reflecting good, fair and poor prognoses.

Mitotic rate

Mitotic rate is recorded by square millimetre. If it is greater than 6 mm^2, the prognosis is poor.

EVOLUTION OF SURGICAL TREATMENT

The surgical treatment of a primary cutaneous malignant melanoma is controversial and it is useful to trace its evolution.

William Norris recorded that, in 1817, he had removed a primary melanoma between the umbilicus and pubis 'with the knife' and that it recurred in the scar in less than six weeks. In 1857, when reporting 'eight cases of melanosis', Norris described a woman aged 26 years with a mole between the shoulders. Her brother had run 'a pair of scissors through it with the hope of removing it'. But three months later, it began to grow and Norris removed 'all the disease with abundance of the surrounding tissue. The wound healed satisfactorily and there was no return of the disease within eight years. So there is good historical evidence extending for over 150 years that melanoma recurs locally after minimal excision (and apparently shave biopsy), but may not recur when an 'abundance' of normal surrounding skin is removed.

Sampson Handley, because of his writings in 1907, has been given the credit (or blame) for advocating wide excision (5 cm margin) and routine regional lymphadenectomy. Pringle, in 1908, went further and advocated wide local excision, regional lymphadenectomy and removal of skin and subcutaneous tissues between primary tumour and the nodes.

This radical approach to melanoma extended well into the 1960s and the writings of Pack *et al*[19] from the USA, Sir Stanford Cade[20] and Petersen *et al*[21] from England and Grete Olsen[22] from Denmark added great authority to this approach. Many examples of recurrence and death after conservative surgery were given.

In the 1960s, pathologists started to take a renewed interest in the study of melanoma. Mehnert and Heard[23] proposed in 1965 that melanoma should be staged according to depth of invasion and claimed that the staging gave a guide to prognosis. A group of Australian pathologists met in 1966 in Brisbane and produced a terminology and classification for moles and melanoma[24]. Clark *et al*[10] introduced the microanatomical levels and Breslow[11] introduced his measurement of tumour thickness. These studies of the pathology made surgeons think about and question the dogma of routine radical surgery for all melanomas.

Public and professional education, initiated in 1963 by the Queensland Melanoma Project[25] had the effect of bringing patients to their doctors at an earlier biological stage (i.e. with thinner melanomas) than previously. This has prompted much discussion in the last decade about how widely individual melanomas should be excised.

In contrast to the 5 cm or more margin accepted up to the mid-1960s, Ackerman and Scheiner[26] state categorically that wide excisions are unnecessary and unjustified for primary melanomas of any thickness. They say the surgeon should excise only what he clinically judges to be the entire neoplasm and little more than that. In short, they claim that surgery for primary melanomas should be no different from that for any other primary neoplasm of the skin (for example BCC).

Sondergaard and Schou[27] report, after analysis of their series, that the width of excision margins has no effect on survival. Other authors report that while the incidence of local recurrence is low

(4.5%),[28] the percentage of local recurrence increases with greater thickness of tumour and decreases with wide margins of excision. The problem about local or regional recurrence is that, in many cases, it is followed by disseminated melanomas. Even if it is not followed by dissemination, local or regional recurrence often poses great problems for both the surgeon and the patient in its management. Many experienced surgeons are unwilling at present to advise and practise excision with narrow margins for all melanomas. Melanoma is a serious cutaneous melanoma, immeasurably worse than BCC or SCC with fatal consequences in many cases if it recurs. Until properly designed randomized trials, carried out and followed up in large numbers over at least 10 years, show that excision margins are inconsequential, I believe the margins, especially for thick lesions, should not be skimped. The addition of 2–3 cm of skin is not a major problem in most surgical excisions, and the cosmetic effect is usually quite acceptable. It is conceded that a skin graft with a contour defect is not as cosmetically acceptable as a linear scar. I have a philosophy that 'it is better to have a large scar than a small tombstone'.

PRACTICAL CONSIDERATIONS IN LOCAL SURGICAL TREATMENT

In the local surgical treatment of a primary melanoma, the surgeon aims to excise as little normal tissue as possible, but as much as is necessary to ensure a cure. Surgeons differ, as pointed out above, about the required margin of excision. I believe that there is no absolute answer that applies to each case. In some instances, the melanoma will be over-treated, and in others under-treated. As the consequences of undertreatment may be fatal, I have a bias towards over-treatment. I believe my patients would prefer a large excision, if there was any risk at all that a smaller excision would be associated with recurrence. It must be realized that melanoma is not a uniform disease. Many thin melanomas are highly curable, whatever the margin of excision. Many advanced melanomas are incurable, whatever is done. However, I believe that, in an appreciable number of patients, appropriate treatment will cure whereas inappropriate treatment will not.

The local treatment for a patient with a melanoma should be individualized. The surgeon will make his judgement of appropriate treatment on his past experience with the disease and his knowledge of the literature. Let me say clearly that I believe the statement that surgery for a melanoma should be no different from that, for example, for a basal cell carcinoma is nonsense.

To make any sort of rational decision, the surgeon should consider the factors that influence the prognosis. These have been outlined above.

When the prognostic factors are favourable

In thin lesions (less than 0.76 mm) that show no evidence of local regression, or in patients with melanoma *in situ* or invading only to level II, a margin of 2 cm is usually adequate and can be less on the face (5 mm). A skin graft is hardly ever indicated in such thin lesions. It is worth noting that the Queensland Melanoma Project has records of five patients who have died, and eleven who developed lymph node metastases from primary cutaneous melanomas less than 0.76 mm thick. Consequently, these lesions should not be treated casually.

For thicker lesions (greater than 0.76 mm and less than 1.5 mm) and those invading to level III and beyond

In such cases I advise excision with a margin between 2 and 5 cm, depending on the histogenetic type, the sex of the patient, the anatomic site of the tumour, the presence or absence of ulceration and the previous treatment. I usually take the maximum margin that allows primary closure without a skin graft.

When the prognostic factors are very unfavourable (thickness greater than 1.5 mm or invading to level IV or beyond)

Under such conditions, especially where the melanoma is situated in an unpredictable lymph node area, I have no hesitation in performing a 5 cm margin of excision, and covering the defect with a split skin graft. In spite of Olsen's work, I usually include the deep fascia in the excision, to reduce the risk of cutting too close to the deep surface of the tumour. While the size of resection margins may not correlate with length of survival, I cannot bring myself to treat a high-risk melanoma with a minimal excision. When a skin graft is necessary, I prefer a split skin graft to a rotation flap in most cases, for two reasons: (1) if a recurrence develops, it is easier to diagnose with a split skin graft than a flap, and (2) a rotation flap has the potential for spreading any residual tumour cells via the lymphatics. In general, many lesions on the face, especially lentigo maligna melanomas, may be excised with only 5 mm margin. Subungual melanoma and acral lentiginous melanomas often require amputation of the digit involved.

Regional lymph nodes

Lymph nodes clinically involved with melanoma are round and are usually greater than 1 cm in diameter. They are firm and rubbery, rather than hard. They are rarely fixed to surrounding structures. Nodes that are clinically involved or suspected to be so should be excised by block dissection, where possible in continuity with excision of a primary melanoma. The prognosis depends on the number of metastatic nodes involved.

Elective lymphadenectomy of clinically normal nodes remains a controversial subject. However, if it were of overwhelming value it would be now universally accepted. I believe there is no place for its routine adoption. Microstaging of the primary melanoma, by measuring the thickness and estimating the level of dermal invasion, is of help in indicating the necessity or otherwise of lymphadenectomy. Patients with melanomas 0.76 mm or less thick, with no signs of local regression or with melanomas invading only to levels I or II, never need elective dissection. Elective dissection may well be indicated for a large ulcerated tumour greater than 1.5 mm thick in the immediate vicinity of or reasonably close to a predictable lymph node area. There is no substitute for surgical judgement and experience in making these decisions. Melanomas greater than 4 mm thick have a high incidence of distant metastases and, while elective dissection may reveal occult metastases, the long-term survival rate may not be altered.

FOLLOW-UP

Regular follow-up examinations of the patient after primary surgical treatment are essential. In general, I see patients every three months for two years, every four months for the next year, every six months for the fourth and fifth years and yearly thereafter. Particular attention is paid to the original scar, and to the regional nodes. If these become enlarged and are suspected of harbouring metastases, I advise lymphadenectomy without preliminary biopsy. There is a risk of about 4% of a patient developing a secondary primary melanoma and at every examination the whole body should be inspected for suspicious moles. I do not practise routine X-rays or scans in the follow-up of patients.

RECURRENT DISEASE

Isolated regional perfusion has been found useful for patients who develop regional 'in-transit' metastases, but is not advised as primary treatment. Amputation of the limb is occasionally indicated, as a palliative manoeuvre, for a fungating recurrence in the limb. Radiotherapy has a small place in treatment. It should be considered as a second line of treatment when the patient is unfit for surgery or the tumour is too far advanced for surgery. Tumours are occasionally radiosensitive.

Where a metastasis can be excised surgically, it should be excised. Some patients have had long survival following removal of a solitary pulmonary or cerebral metastasis.

When melanoma is widely disseminated, the patient should be considered for treatment with DTIC (imidazole carboxamide) and interferon. Workers at the Princess Alexandra Hospital have reported some good remissions.

SURVIVAL DATA[29]

The actuarial survival data, at five and ten years, for 1441 stage I melanoma patients treated in Queensland between July, 1963 and December 1969 are shown in Table 2.1. The data are subdivided for sex, site of primary tumour, tumour thickness and presence or absence of ulceration.

TABLE 2.1 Actuarial survival data for 1441 stage 'I' melanoma patients treated in Queensland between 1963 and 1969

	Survival rates (%)	
	5-Year	*10-Year*
All patients	85%	80%
Male patients	79%	72%
Female patients	90%	86%
Primary site		
Lower limb	90%	86%
Upper limb	90%	89%
Head & neck	83%	76%
Trunk	79%	71%
Tumour thickness		
< 0.76 mm	97%	95%
0.76 – 1.49 mm	92%	87%
1.50 – 2.49 mm	83%	76%
2.50 – 3.99 mm	77%	63%
> 4.00 mm	48%	40%
Ulceration		
Yes	68%	60%
No	91%	87%

PUBLIC AND PROFESSIONAL EDUCATION

From the commencement of the Queensland Melanoma Project in 1963, much attention has been paid to public and professional education. Because of the high incidence of skin cancer and melanoma in the state, the Queensland Cancer Fund and the Division of Health Education & Information of the Queensland Health Department set out to educate the public on the early signs of skin cancer and its relation to exposure to sun, as well as on the danger signs in a mole. This programme utilizes lectures, discussions and films led by specially trained nurses. It is directed at primary and secondary school children, at community groups (e.g., Rotary clubs), at industry and business houses and at public forums. This aim is to develop a sensible attitude to skin care and protection while recognizing the desire of people to enjoy Queensland's wonderful climate. The opportunity is taken to put skin cancer, melanoma and other common cancers into proper perspective. Articles appear in the daily newspapers and the educational message is promoted on radio and television.

Many pamphlets and posters have been produced. These are displayed in shops, pharmacies, libraries, doctor's surgeries and other public places. The brand names of the sunscreens providing maximum protection against ultraviolet rays are constantly publicized. Individuals are advised to apply sunscreens with a skin protection factor (SPF) greater than 15. The public are advised to 'slip on a shirt, slop on a sunscreen and slap on a hat'. The Premier has publicized a wide-brimmed Joh hat. The public are advised of the dangers of exposure to sun between 11am and 2pm. In the melanoma field, a bookmark and a cartoon indicating the danger signs in a mole have proved effective. The members of the Queensland Melanoma Project have always made themselves available to the media – usually anonymously. They are commonly the source of articles on melanoma that appear in the local and national press each year. On every possible occasion, the danger signs of moles are stressed. Whatever else is said or written, the public are told to consult their doctor if a mole undergoes any unusual change. In recent years, dermatologists have organized a Skin Cancer Awareness Week and free clinics have been set up to diagnose suspicious skin lesions. Perhaps even more attention has been paid by the Queensland Melanoma Project to professional education. A colour film with sound has been produced and is shown to medical students, nurses and allied health professionals. Illustrated colour pamphlets on the differential diagnosis and management of pigmented skin tumours are supplied free of charge to medical students and practitioners. Scientific displays have been mounted and audiovisual programmes have been developed. Throughout the year, members of the Project lecture to students and at postgraduate meetings locally, nationally and internationally. More than seventy publications on various aspects of melanoma have appeared in scientific journals. Our principal pathologist, Dr. J. Little, provides a free consultative service for pathologists throughout the state and nation for the interpretation of difficult pigmented cell tumours. It is of interest that, despite the increasing incidence of the disease in Queensland, the mortality from melanoma in Queensland has remained steady. This is in contrast to the incidence and mortality in every other Australian state, both of which have risen[30]. It seems reasonable to claim that melanoma is one cancer for which public and professional education has improved the prognosis.

REFERENCES

1. Norris, W. (1820). Case of fungoid disease. *Edinburgh Medical & Surgical J.* **16**, 562
2. Davis, N.C. and McLeod, G.R. (1985). The history of melanoma from Hunter to Handley (1787–1907) In: Balch, C.M. and Milton, G.W., (eds.) Cutaneous Melanoma, p.1. (Philadelphia: Lippincott)
3. Lee, J.A.H. (1983). Epidemiology of malignant melanoma: 10 years progress. In Mackie, R. (ed.) Vol. 6, pp.1–21. Pigment Cell (Basel: Karger)
4. Little, J.H., Holt, J. and Davis, N. (1980). Changing epidemiology of malignant melanoma in Queensland. *Med. J. Aust.*, **1**, 66–9
5. Davis, N.C. (1976). Cutaneous melanoma: The Queensland Experience. *Curr. Prob. Surg.* **13**, 1–63
6. Davis, N.C. (1982). Malignant melanoma: clinical presentation and differential diagnosis. In Emmett, A.J.J. and O'Rourke, M.G.E.(eds.) *Malignant Skin Tumours*, pp. 107–116. (Edinburgh: Churchill Livingstone)
7. Ackerman, A.B. and Su, W.P.D. (1979). The histology of cutaneous malignant melanoma. In Kopf, A.W., Bart, R.S., Rodriguez-Sains, R.S. and Ackerman, A.B. (eds). *Malignant Melanoma*, pp. 25–147. (New York: Mason)
8. Elder, D.E., Greene, M.H., Bondi, E.E. and Clark, W.H. (1981). Acquired melanotic nevi and melanoma: the dysplastic nevus syndrome. In Ackerman,

A.B. (ed.) *Pathology of Malignant Melanoma*. pp.185–215. (New York: Masson)

9. Dixon, S.L. and Ackerman, A.B. (1985) Some observations, reflections and questions about dysplastic nevi, *Am. J. Dermatopathol.*, **7**, **A** 17–25 (Supplement)
10. Clark, W., From, L., Bernandino, E. and Mihm, M. (1969). The histogenesis and biological behaviour of primary human malignant melanoma of the skin. *Cancer Res.*, **29**, 705–27
11. Breslow, A. (1970). Thickness, cross sectional areas and depth of invasion in the prognosis of cutaneous melanoma. *Ann. Surg.*, **172**, 902–8
12. McGovern, V.J., Cochran, A.J., Van der Esch, E.P., Little, J.H. and MacLennon, R. (1986). The classification of malignant melanoma, its histological reporting and registration: a revision of the 1972 Sydney Classification. *Pathology*, **18**, 12–21
13 Little, J.H. and Davis, N.C. (1974). Frozen section diagnosis of suspected malignant melanoma of the skin. *Cancer*, **34**, 1163
14. Balch, C.M., Soong, S.J., Shaw, H.M. and Milton, G.W. (1985). An analysis of prognostic factors in 4000 patients with cutaneous melanoma. In Balch, C.M. and Milton G.W. (eds.) *Cutaneous Melanoma.* Clinical Management and Treatment Results Worldwide., pp.321–52. (Philadelphia: Lippincott)
15. Day, C.L., Mihm, M.C., Soher, A.J. *et al.* (1982). Prognostic factors for melanoma patients with lesions 0.76 – 1.69 mm in thickness. *Ann. Surg.*, **195**, 30–4
16. Woods, J.E., Soule, E.H., and Greagan, E.T. (1983). Metastasis and death in patients with thin melanomas (less than 0.76 mm). *Ann. Surg.*, **198**, 63–4
17. Ackerman, A.B. (1980). Malignant melanoma: a unifying concept. *Hum. Pathol.*, **11**, 591–5
18. Schmoeckel, C. and Braun-Falco, O. (1978). Prognostic index in malignant melanoma. *Arch. Dermatol.* **114**, 871–3
19. Pack, G.T., Gerber, D.N. and Scharnagel, I.M. (1952). End results of the treatment of malignant melanoma: a report of 1190 cases. *Ann. Surg.* **136**, 904–11
20. Cade, S. (1961). Malignant melanoma. *Ann. R. Coll. Surg. Engl.* **23**, 331–66
21. Petersen, N.C., Bodenham, D.C. and Lloyd, O.C. (1962). Malignant melanomas of the skin. *Br. J. Plast. Surg.*, **15**, 97–116
22. Olsen, G. (1966). *The malignant melanoma of the skin.* (Copenhagen: The Finsen Institute and Radium Centre)
23. Mehnert, J.H. and Heard, J.L. (1965). Staging of malignant melanoma by depth of invasion. *Am. J. Surg.*, **110**, 168–76
24. McGovern, V.J., Caldwell, R.A., Duncan, C.A. *et al.* (1967). Moles and malignant melanoma: terminology and classification. *Med. J. Aust.*, **1**, 123–4
25. Davis, N.C. and Herron, J.J. (1966). Queensland Melanoma Project:- organisation and a plea for comparable surveys. *Med. J. Aust.*, **1**, 643–4
26. Ackerman, A.B. and Scheiner, A.M. (1983). A critique of surgical practice in excisions of primary cutaneous malignant melanoma. *Hum. Pathol.*, **14,** 743–4
27. Sondergaard, K. and Schou, G. (1985). Biopsy and optimal size of margins of resection of primary cutaneous malignant melanomas. *Am. J. Dermatopathol.*, **7**, 127–9 (Supplement)
28. Veronisi, U. and Cascinelli, N. (1985). Margins of resection of malignant melanomas that are less than the hitherto conventional 'wide and deep' margins

are not advisable as yet. *Am. J. Dermatopathol.*, **7**, 123–6 (Supplement)

29. McLeod, G.R., Davis, N.C., Little, J.H., Green, A. and Chant, D. (1985). Melanoma in Queensland, Australia: experience of the Queensland Melanoma Project. In Balch, C.M. and Milton, G.W. (eds.) *Cutaneous Melanoma. Clinical Management and Treatment Results Worldwide*, pp. 379–87 (Philadelphia: Lippincott).
30. Armstrong, B.K., Holman, C.D., Ford, J.M. and Woodings, T.L. (1982). Trend in melanoma incidence and mortality in Australia. In Magnus, K. (ed.) *Trends in Cancer Incidence*.,pp. 399–417. (Washington: Hemisphere)

3

THE DIAGNOSIS AND MANAGEMENT OF CUTANEOUS LYMPHOMAS

M. F. SPITTLE

The diseases presenting as cutaneous lymphoma are fascinating, showing a wide diversity of natural history, clinical appearances and response to treatment. These diseases are rare, but can often confidently be clinically segregated into the varying types of cutaneous lymphoma. The clinical and histopathological classifications have been facilitated by recent advances in immunocytochemistry.

Mycosis fungoides is the most commonly occurring cutaneous lymphoma. This is considered[1] to be of T-cell origin and in general has a protracted course, being confined to the skin for a large part of the natural history of the disease. The Sézary syndrome, dissimilar clinically, is the erythrodermic variant that exhibits a number of circulating atypical mononuclear cells in the blood and is generally less amenable to treatment.

The B-cell lymphomas present a varied and different clinical appearance in the skin and may be part of widespread non-Hodgkin's lymphoma involving bone marrow and lymph nodes. Attempts to classify non-Hodgkin's lymphoma have been numerous and there are several well-known classifications in current use. The morphological and immunological features of the malignant cells in the skin are usually similar to those found in nodes and extranodal sites[2].

The management of the two major forms of cutaneous lymphoma differs widely. Staging procedures are carried out in patients both with B-cell and with T-cell lymphomas, but the demonstration of widespread extracutaneous involvement is more common in the B-cell variant. This dictates that the management of these patients is usually by chemotherapy, to which the initial response is often dramatic; however, the long-term prognosis is poor. In contrast, patients with cutaneous T-cell lymphomas have minimal response to chemotherapy and therefore the mainstays of active specific management are PUVA therapy, topical nitrogen mustard, superficial radiotherapy and electron-beam treatment[3]. The diagnosis and management of lymphocytoma cutis and lymphomatoid papulosis will be described.

MYCOSIS FUNGOIDES

History

In 1806 Alibert[4] described the disease he termed mycosis fungoides in a patient with a skin rash, who subsequently developed skin tumours from which he died. Mycotic diseases were not known at that time and the term mycosis fungoides was designated to describe the tumours as mushrooms on the skin. The 'Maladie d'Alibert' was more fully described by Bazin[5] in 1870 when the three stages of the classical disease were recognized. The slow progression of the non-specific pre-mycotic phase, through the infiltrating plaque stage to the evolution of tumours, constitutes the classical form of the disease. However, a *tumeur d'emblée* variant was described in 1885 by Vidal and Brocq[6] with rapid development of tumours and with little background patterning of the skin. Besnier and Hallopeau[7] identified the erythrodermic phase and poikiloderma atrophicans vasculare was also described in association with mycosis fungoides. In poikiloderma atrophicans vasculare, patches of atrophy, pigmentation and telangiectasia are seen in association with the classical mycosis fungoides lesions, which may be particularly slowly progressive. The *in situ* variant or Pagetoid reticulosis was designated by Worringer and Kolopp[8] and is typically limited to superficial scaly patches of disease affecting the extremities of younger patients. It is rarely associated with lymph node involvement. Occasionally this variant may progress to classical widespread mycosis fungoides.

Sézary[9] recognized the syndrome of erythroderma, enlarged peripheral lymph nodes and circulating large mononuclear cells in 1938. Patients with the widespread erythrodermic form of mycosis fungoides may be difficult to differentiate clinically from those with Sézary syndrome, although pruritus is a less important early symptom in mycosis fungoides.

The mycosis cells found in the dermis of patients with mycosis fungoides are noted to be similar to the atypical circulating cells of the Sézary syndrome. These cells are also occasionally found in the peripheral blood of mycosis fungoides patients. The Lutzner[10] or Sézary cell is characterized as a T-cell of the helper CD4-positive phenotype. The variants of mycosis fungoides, and the Sézary syndrome are now collectively described as cutaneous T-cell lymphoma (CTCL)[11] and this collective heading enables the disease to be considered within the broader discipline of oncology.

Incidence

Cutaneous T-cell lymphoma is a rare disease seen less frequently than Hodgkin's disease; it exhibits a male predominance and, although all age groups can be affected, the majority of these patients are in the age range 40–70 years. No cause has been found, although the association with workers in the chemical and dye industries is noted, as in other lymphomas[12]. Prognosis is variable, but usually good (9–10 years). Although some series of cases from America have a shorter median survival, the European experience is of a relatively benign disease with a long natural history that may depend on the accurate diagnosis of the long pre-mycotic period.

Pathology and immunology

The histopathological features of the cutaneous lesions of mycosis fungoides may vary from patient to patient and with the stage of the disease. The characteristic appearances seen in biopsies from early and plaque-stage disease are a band-like cellular infiltrate in the upper dermis with varying degrees of epidermotropism. The dermal infiltrate consists largely of mononuclear cells, with a variable proportion of histiocytes, eosinophils and other inflammatory cells. A proportion of the mononuclear cells in the dermal infiltrate and those colonizing the epidermis have hyperchromatic and convoluted or cerebriform nuclei. These cells are sometimes referred to as mycosis cells and immunohistochemically are usually of the CD4 (T-helper cell) phenotype. In the advanced stages of mycosis fungoides the dermal infiltrate tends to be more dense and to extend deeply. Epidermotropism is often lost and histopathological differentiation from other forms of lymphoma may be difficult.

A detailed discussion of the immunology and histogenesis of mycosis fungoides is beyond the scope of this chapter. However, it is clear that, as well as T-lymphocytes, cells of the histiocyte macrophage series including the Langerhans cells of the epidermis and probably dermal indeterminate cells play an important role in the pathogenesis of the disease. Readers are referred to the excellent review by Norris and LeFeber[13] for further discussion of this topic.

Since the discovery of the RNA retrovirus, antibodies to this specific virus have been found in the sera of patients with cutaneous T-cell lymphoma. In one such group of patients, a cutaneous T-cell lymphoma associated with hypercalcaemia and bony involvement has been characterized as HTLV1 disease[14]. Common membrane antigens have been noted from patients with CTCL and AIDS patients affected with the HIV retrovirus[15]. There is therefore suggestive evidence of an aetiological association between cutaneous T-cell lymphoma and virus[16].

Staging

There have been several attempts to stage mycosis fungoides in a similar way to other lymphomas, but the importance of the extent of the disease in the skin, both in depth of infiltration and in area, is then underestimated. In 1978 a workshop on cutaneous T-cell lymphoma held at the National Cancer Institute agreed on the modified staging system shown below in Table 3.1.

TABLE 3.1 Tumour, nodes, metastases (TNM) classification of cutaneous T-cell lymphoma (CTCL)

Classification	*Description*
T: skin[a]	
T_0	Clinically and/or histopathologically suspicious lesions
T_1	Limited plaques, papules, or eczematoid patches covering less than 10% of the skin surface
T_2	Generalized plaques, papules, or erythematous patches covering 10% or more of the skin surface
T_3	Tumours, one or more
T_4	Generalized erythroderma
N: lymph nodes[b]	
N_0	No clinically or palpably abnormal peripheral lymph nodes; pathology negative for CTCL
N_1	Clinical abnormal peripheral lymph nodes; pathology negative for CTCL
N_2	No clinically abnormal peripheral lymph nodes; pathology positive for CTCL
N_3	Clinically abnormal peripheral lymph nodes; pathology positive for CTCL
B: peripheral blood	
B_0	Atypical circulating cells not present, or less than 5%
B_1	Atypical circulating cells present in 5% or more; record total white blood cell count and total lymphocyte counts and number of atypical cells/100 lymphocytes.
M: visceral organs	
M_0	No involvement of visceral organs
M_1	Visceral involvement (must have confirmation of pathology and organ involved should be specified)

a Pathology of T1-4 is diagnostic of a CTCL. When characteristics of more than one T exist, both are recorded and the highest is used for staging, e.g., T^4.
b The number of sites of abnormal nodes are recorded, e.g., cervical (left + right), axillary (left + right), inguinal (left + right), epitrochlear, submandibular, submaxillary

Clinical course

A patient with mycosis fungoides may well have complained of a skin rash for many years prior to diagnosis. It is common for the patient to have been considered to have unresponsive eczema or psoriasis prior to a biopsy being taken. During this phase, the disease is banal, usually presenting as superficial scaly, erythematous, irregular areas with patches of spared normal skin (Figure 3.1). Where disease is not widespread, it most commonly affects the buttocks and breasts, with the face and extremities frequently being spared. Although the disease may progress more rapidly, particularly in the elderly, on first diagnosis there are usually few infiltrated patches and lymphadenopathy is not common on presentation. However, when widespread, ulcerated and tumour-stage disease is seen there is frequent lymphadenopathy, particularly in the groins and axillae. Unlike Hodgkin's disease, where nodes become involved in a stepwise movement, nodes involved with mycosis fungoides are peripheral and progress centripetally. Follicular mucinosis may occur and, if on the scalp, usually as part of tumour-stage disease, the destruction of hair follicles may cause permanent alopecia.

On diagnosis, the patient should be staged and the type and distribution of skin lesions should be mapped. Although physical exami-

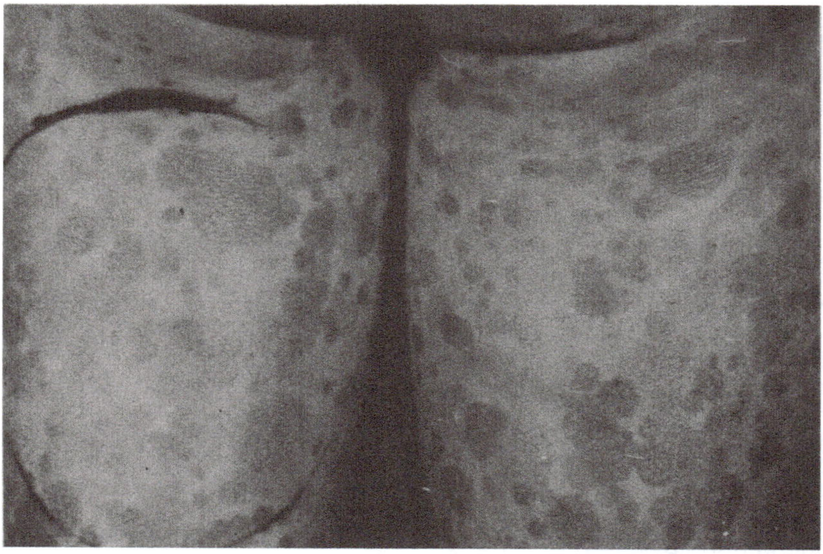

FIGURE 3.1 Widespread superficial mycosis fungoides. Note the different shape and shades of the lesions and the spared patches

nation will frequently show enlarged nodes, there is no reliable test of involvement with mycosis fungoides other than biopsy. Lymphangiogram and CT scans have been performed extensively, but show the typical peripheral enlarged nodes frequently seen in skin disease without giving an indication of whether they are due to infection, dermatopathic changes or invasion with mycosis fungoides[17]. A node biopsy therefore is an important adjunct to staging. Dermatopathic changes are associated with a poorer prognosis than when the node is normal, although frank mycosis fungoides may not be seen[18]. A bone marrow examination is mandatory in all lymphomas, but this is not usually helpful in mycosis fungoides. Involvement is rare other than with cells that are passing through the bone marrow.

Although mycosis fungoides may affect any internal organ, this is unusual at presentation. Visualization of the liver and spleen as a base-line investigation, by either ultrasound or CT scan may be performed. Full blood count and differential and search for Sézary cells are also important.

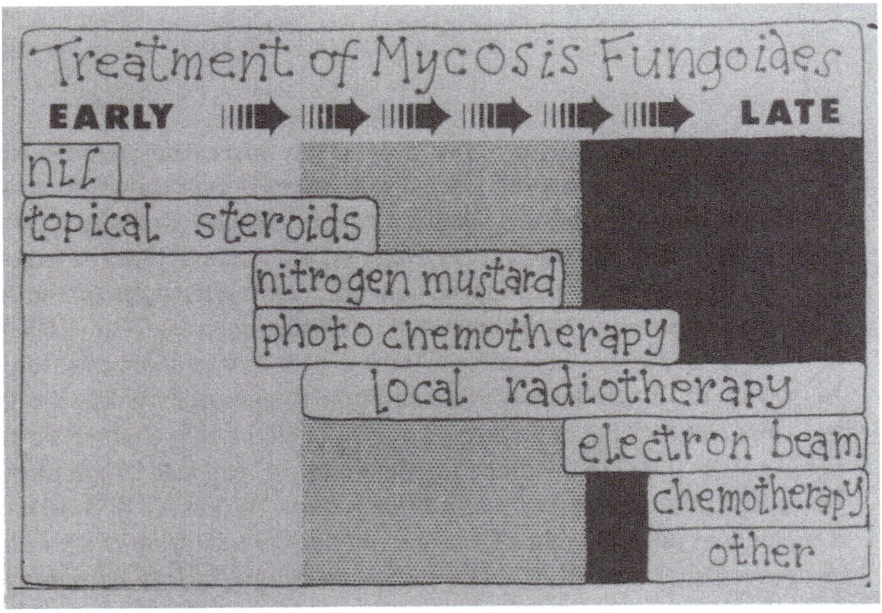

FIGURE 3.2 Treatment of mycosis fungoides. (Courtesy of Dr. N.P. Smith.)

Treatment (Figure 3.2)

Symptomatic

In the early stage classical disease, when superficial plaques are confined to the buttock area or are only a little more widespread, treatment is rarely required. If the skin becomes sore, the use of an emulsifying ointment in the bath or a non-steroid moisturizer is often all that is required.

Symptomatic lesions may be controlled for long periods by the application of dilute hydrocortisone ointment or other mild steroid. The occasional pruritus can be treated with antihistamines, which are especially useful at night. The anxiety and depression associated with a chronic skin condition can often be relieved by specific medication and counselling of the patient about the nature of the disease underlining the availability of more active treatment should the lesions become progressive. Patients with widespread symptomatic involvement can be treated either by PUVA therapy or by topical nitrogen mustard.

PUVA (Figure 3.3)

PUVA therapy has become available in an increasing number of large dermatological centres since 1978, when it was shown to control superficial mycosis fungoides[19]. Patients receive 8-methoxypsoralen in a dose depending on their weight, two hours prior to exposure of the total body to long-wavelength ultraviolet light of the A spectrum (wavelength approximately 350 nanometres). The PUVA exposure is expressed in joules. Starting with only a short exposure, the treatment time is increased on subsequent occasions until a mild erythema occurs. Treatment may initially be given two or three times weekly. As the skin develops pigmentation in response to the ultraviolet light, the treatment times are increased. When the disease has come under control and has flattened out and no new lesions are seen to be occurring, the PUVA treatment can be given less frequently. Initially this may be reduced to once weekly or once a fortnight. When the patient's skin is clear it can then be discontinued until such time as the lesions recur, when the PUVA therapy can be restarted.

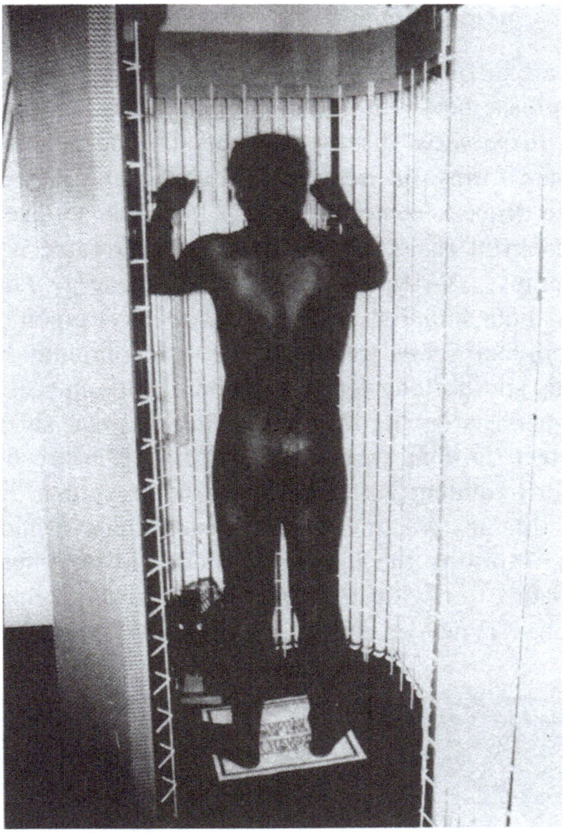

FIGURE 3.3 Patient undergoing PUVA therapy

There is evidence to show that discontinuing the PUVA when the patient's skin is clear and restarting when necessary is as effective in controlling the disease as long-term maintainance PUVA[20].

Side-effects of psoralen tablets are few; some patients exhibit mild nausea, headache or stinging of the skin. Since 8-methoxypsoralen sensitizes the patient to ultraviolet light, to avoid the production of cataracts the patient should wear sunglasses for the remainder of the day. Patients are usually treated with PUVA in a standing position and smaller machines are available to treat areas such as hands and feet. During the PUVA therapy, the eyes are protected with goggles and the patient is positioned so that the radiation can reach all parts of the body.

Superficial X-ray treatment

Some areas are difficult to treat with PUVA - the perineum, under the feet, in the crease below the buttocks, in the hair and behind the eye shields. In these sites, disease may persist and become thickened, needing other forms of treatment. These and other patches of tumour-stage disease, occurring in a patient whose disease is otherwise under control on PUVA therapy, can be treated with low-voltage radiotherapy. X-rays in the 80–120 kV energy range are most appropriate. Four hundred centigrays (400 cGy) given on two occasions is usually sufficient treatment to cause complete disappearance of the lesions and no long-term radiation change in the skin. Where the disease persists on the eyelids, an internal eye shield of lead is used to protect the lens from the radiation. Disease becoming too infiltrated for treatment with PUVA on the scalp is a difficult problem, as radiotherapy treatment will cause temporary alopecia of the treated sites. Cutting the hair very short and treatment with P-32 strontium plaque[21] or with topical nitrogen mustard, may be used in this situation. However, if the disease goes untreated, follicular

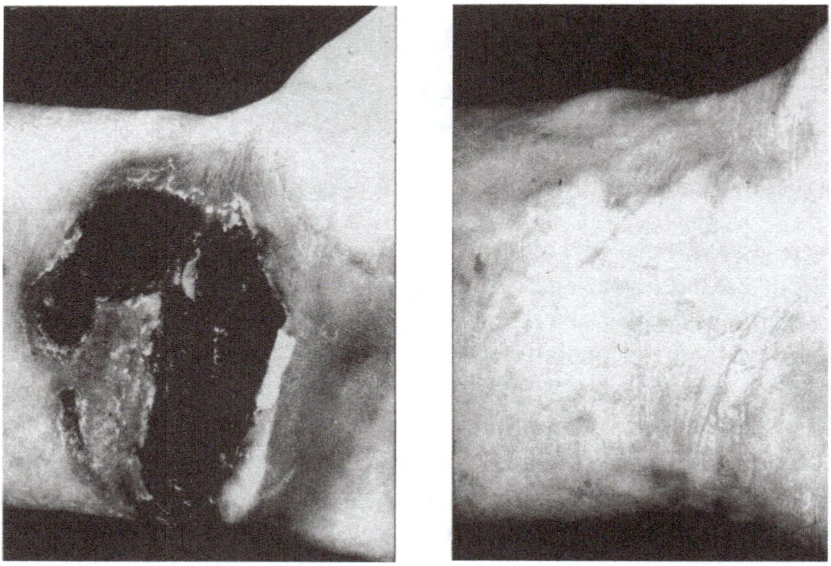

FIGURE 3.4 Mycosis fungoides. Before and after low-voltage radiotherapy

mucinosis and subsequent permanent alopecia will occur owing to destruction of the hair follicles.

Occasionally, patches of infiltrated mycosis fungoides may occur in patients with early disease before definitive treatment is necessary. Low-voltage radiotherapy of that site gives an excellent local response (Figures 3.4 and 3.5).

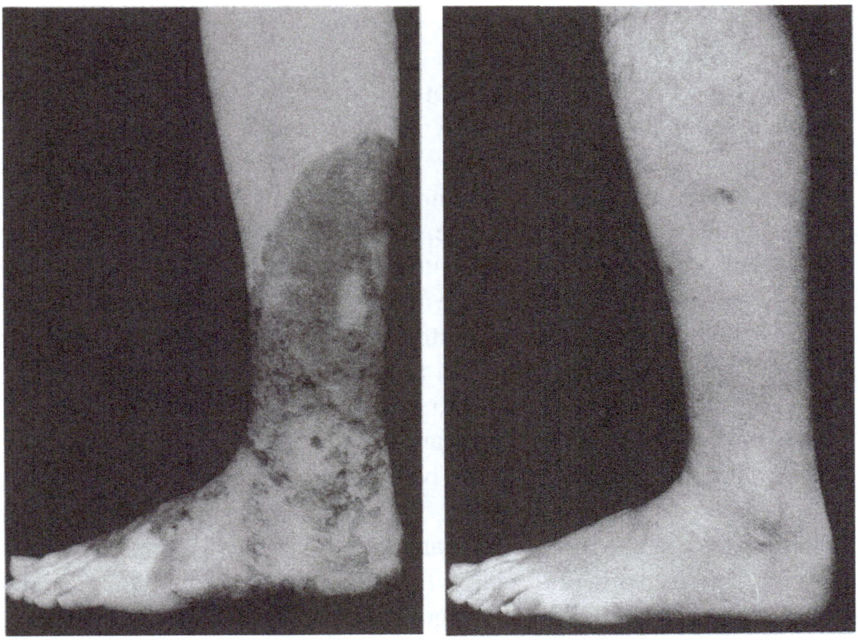

FIGURE 3.5 Worringer and Kolopp variant of mycosis fungoides (a) before and (b) after low-voltage radio-therapy

Topical nitrogen mustard

Topical nitrogen mustard therapy is frequently used to treat superficial mycosis fungoides[22] where PUVA centres are not geographically convenient. A 10 mg vial of mustine is diluted in 50 ml of tap water and, using the gloved hand, may be spread daily over the skin of the patient. Sensitization is common, occurring in about 30% of the cases, but this may be overcome by increasing the dilution of the nitrogen mustard until it is tolerated and then slowly increasing the concentration again. Nitrogen mustard may also be put in an emulsifying ointment that is easier to manage and does not accumulate so readily in skin creases. There is also less chance of sensitization. The use of topical nitrogen mustard is particularly favoured for patients for whom access to a PUVA unit is not possible.

Electron beam therapy

Tumour-stage disease that cannot be controlled either by PUVA or by occasional local radiotherapy to ulcerated lesions may be controlled by electron-beam therapy[23]. A superficial electron beam has a limited-depth dose in tissue and no unwanted radiation need be given to the tissues underlying the dermis. Whole-skin irradiation may therefore be given without unwanted effects on the blood count, bone marrow or lungs. Using a large field from a linear accelerator and placing the patient in several treatment positions relative to the beam, the whole skin may be treated in as homogenous a manner as possible. Although many schedules are described, we use 300 cGy given twice a week to eight fields in an attempt to treat the whole body. This treatment is continued for five weeks giving a total dose to the skin of 3000 cGy (Figure 3.6). Following this treatment, the skin becomes red and may desquamate locally at the site of infiltrated lesions. Apart from this generalized soreness, the patient has few other symptoms. The blood count is rarely affected by the treatment. Some late pigmentation may occur. There is total, usually temporary, alopecia in all areas and occasionally a transient lower limb lymphoedema may persist. It is rare that a patient does not totally clear of disease after this treatment. Whole-skin electron beam therapy to this dose cannot be repeated. Late skin change producing telangectasia, which occurs to some extent in about half of the patients, denotes that tolerance has been reached. In some centres, electron beam treatment is used earlier in the progress of the disease in an attempt to cure patients. Although long remissions are seen, these are difficult to assess in a disease with a long and variable natural history. When electron-beam therapy is relegated to treat advanced disease, then, once clearance has been obtained, maintenance therapy with PUVA is important.

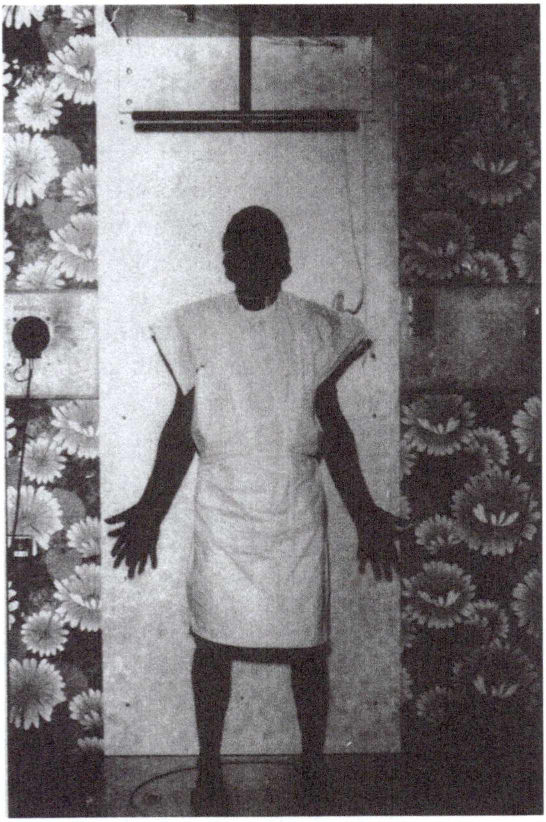

FIGURE 3.6 Patient receiving whole-skin electron-beam therapy – one of eight positions

The general philosophy of management of mycosis fungoides is slightly different on either side of the Atlantic. In North America, the emphasis is on radical treatment in an attempt to cure early disease, accepting the slight, but persisting telangectasia that may occur[24]. In Britain, electron-beam treatment is usually reserved until tumour-stage disease has occurred and more conservative treatments have failed (Figure 3.7).

Chemotherapy and immunotherapy

In view of the general philosophy of treatment of mycosis fungoides and the relative chemoresistance of the disease, chemotherapy is relegated to the treatment of advanced tumour-stage disease, that has recurred after electron-beam therapy. There is good evidence (viz. alopecia) that intravenous cytotoxic chemotherapy reaches the skin and lymphomas are in general extremely sensitive to and may be cured by chemotherapy. However, mycosis fungoides has always been an enigma in this respect, with quite inconsistent and short-term response to multi-agent cytotoxic therapy[25]. Regimes including cyclophosphamide, vincristine and steroids, with or without adriamycin, have the best reputation in treatment of this disease. The initial response may be good, but the long-term results are less encouraging. Tolerance of chemotherapy may be poor and care must be taken, especially with the initial course, to support the patient with good general medical care.

The retinoids may be useful in some cases of hypertrophic lichenified mycosis fungoides. Care must be taken with widespread disease

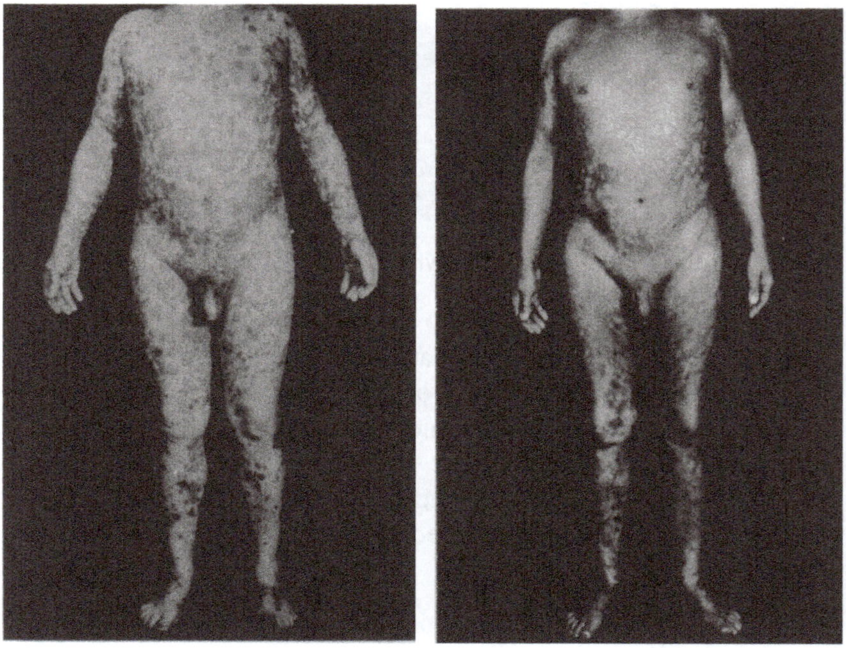

FIGURE 3.7 (a) Before and (b) after whole-skin electron-beam therapy for mycosis fungoides

in atrophic skin, since ulceration may occur. The toxic effects of etretinate include dryness and peeling lips and nose and derangement of liver function.

There are variable results from treatment of mycosis fungoides with interferons and response rates of 60% have been recorded, especially with early-stage disease. The duration of response may be considerable (up to three years), but the side-effects of the interferon must be considered in the light of the many skin treatment modalities available for early-stage disease.

SÉZARY SYNDROME

This variant of CTCL is characterized clinically by erythroderma, generalized lymphadenopathy, pruritus, oedema and hyperkeratosis of the palms and soles. The circulating blood often contains large numbers of large atypical mononuclear cells with deeply cleaved and folded nuclei. This syndrome presents *de novo*, rarely going through the phase of clinical mycosis fungoides. The skin is usually atrophic. Treatment is difficult, as neither PUVA nor electron-beam therapy is generally successful. The course of the disease is variable and response to treatment is correspondingly difficult to assess. Pulsed chlorambucil and steroids may be effective and cause little morbidity. Care must be taken with cytotoxic chemotherapy, as patients with mycosis fungoides and those with Sézary syndrome appear more sensitive to chemotherapy than those with other lymphomas, with frequent massive falls in leucocytes after moderate doses. Although steroids are usually helpful, their withdrawal is often associated with a flare of disease. Retinoids, interferon and leukopheresis have been tried with occasional success. The newer technique of photopheresis may hold hope for these patients[26]. However, the importance of the number of circulating cells is not known, since this varies widely without effecting a change in the clinical condition. Although these cells may be found in the bone marrow, they do not seem to originate there. Sézary cells may occasionally be found circulating in the blood of patients with mycosis fungoides.

B-CELL CUTANEOUS LYMPHOMAS

Pathology

Lymphomas of the B-cell type reflect the multiplicity of B-cells subtypes and their development and function. The clinical diseases produced by these varying clones of lymphoid cells have a different clinical course and hence the nomenclature and classification of the abnormal cells is of prime importance. When these B-cell lymphomas affect the skin, it is usually as part of a systemic lymphoma with lymph node infiltration progressing to bone marrow infiltration[27]. In the rare cases in which the skin is the only manifestation of the B-cell lymphoma at presentation, the disease continues primarily as a skin lymphoma. The histological classifications were initially morphological (Rappaport)[28], but have subsequently become related more to function of B-cell subsets as a result of advances in immunohistochemistry.

Difficulties in the diagnosis of subtypes can usually be resolved by the use of more modern immunological markers, which may be used in sections both of the skin and of the lymph nodes. The typical B-cell pattern of histological involvement of the skin is of aggregates of lymphoid cells sparing the subepidermal or grenz zone. Massive involvement of the appendages and blood vessels is seen. The Lukes and Collins system[29], the Kiel system[30] and that devised by the British Lymphoma Investigation[31] include the functional as well as the morphological element in diagnosis. These several classifications have been found to be consistently reproducible. The non-Hodgkin's lymphoma pathological classification was produced by a working party at the National Cancer Institute in 1982 (see Table 3.2).

Clinical course

In general the B-cell cutaneous lymphoma tends to be more monomorphic than mycosis fungoides and, although it can affect the whole skin, it does not specifically seem to be present on the buttocks in the early stages. There is no scaliness, and the skin appears shiny over the lesions, which are smooth with a relatively sharp edge.

They tend to be brighter rather than dusky red and are usually not itchy. In contrast to cutaneous T-cell lymphoma, the lesions may evolve extremely rapidly, producing gross widespread tumours, especially in the elderly.

Although the prognosis of the lymphoma is dictated by its histological type, all patients with cutaneous lymphoma should be staged. This includes a full clinical examination, blood count with ESR and differential white count, chest X-ray, CT scan of the abdomen and pelvis and bone marrow examination, both aspirate and trephine. This will detect the extent of disease. Patients with B-cell lymphoma are frequently found to have bone marrow involvement. Even if this is not the case, the extreme chemo-sensitivity of this disease, unlike mycosis fungoides, makes chemotherapy the treatment of choice.

TABLE 3.2 Nomenclature proposed by the non-Hodgkin's lymphoma pathological classification project for clinical usage: the working formulation[a]

Type of lymphoma	*Description*
Low-grade lymphomas	Small lymphocytic (consistent with CLL; plasmacytoid)[b]
	Follicular predominantly small cleaved cell (diffuse areas; sclerosis)
	Follicular mixed, small cleaved and large cells (diffuse areas; sclerosis)
Intermediate-grade lymphomas	Follicular predominantly large cell (diffuse areas; sclerosis)
	Diffuse small cleaved cell (sclerosis)
	Diffuse mixed small - and large-cell (sclerosis; epitheloid cell component)
	Diffuse large cell (cleaved cell; non-cleaved cell; sclerosis)
High-grade lymphomas	Large cell immunoblastic (plasmacytoid; clear cell; polymorphous; epitheloid cell component)
	Lymphoblastic (convoluted; non-convoluted)
	Small non-cleaved cell (Burkitt's; follicular areas)

a From The Non-Hodgkin's Lymphoma Pathologic Classification Project

b Additional morphological features not demonstrated to have statistically significant clinical correlations

Treatment

The traditional chemotherapy for the more aggressive non-Hodgkin's lymphomas is an intravenous pulsed multiple agent combination such as CHOP (cyclophosphamide, adriamycin, vincristine and steroids)[32]. This is usually well-tolerated except in the elderly. The patient should be admitted for chemotherapy and a vascular access line may be preferred. It is usual that the patient's disease clears completely after the first or second course of treatment. The chemotherapy should be continued for six or more courses until there has been complete regression. At that stage, the chemotherapy should be discontinued and the patient should be followed up carefully with repeat staging investigations every three to six months. If the disease does not completely clear within two or three courses of chemotherapy, then a further, more aggressive treatment, either with another chemotherapy regime or with high-dose chemotherapy and bone marrow transplantation should be considered. Treatment with monoclonal anti-idiotypic bodies has been tried[33]. The prognosis of the B-cell cutaneous lymphoma is that associated with the morphological type of lymphoma.

With the less aggressive B-cell lymphomas which initially involve the skin, chemotherapy may cause complete regression of the dermatological manifestations and later recurrences may not involve the skin. The aggressive lymphomas, especially the immunoblastic lymphoma, frequently involve the central nervous system and whole-brain irradiation and intrathecal chemotherapy can be given therapeutically or prophylactically. Occasionally, localized ulcerative disease may be irradiated with superficial X-rays. Again, extensive radiosensitive disease may dissappear with three fractions of 300 cGy given at a voltage appropriate to the depth.

LYMPHOCYTOMA CUTIS

Lymphocytoma cutis is an interesting clinical condition and is extremely satisfying to treat, although little is known of its aetiology[34]. Nodules, which may be many or few in number and may vary in size, occur on the face, trunk or back. They are firm and nonulcerated with an obvious edge. The surface is often red and shiny and the size of lesions may vary. Lesions on the back and trunk may coalesce and are neither painful nor itchy. There is no associated lymphadenopathy.

Histologically, an accumulation of lymphocytes is seen high in the dermis which does not extend into the epidermis. The lymphocytes are essentially normal and are usually not associated with other cell types. The term lymphocytoma cutis may include the pseudolymphoma of Spiegler-Fendt and Jessner's lymphocytic infiltrate. It is important to rule out infiltration with malignant lymphoma or the conditions that can look histologically similar, such as an insect bite or angiolymphoid hyperplasia. Immunophenotypically both B and T cells have been found within these collections of lymphocytes and it may be that the condition is the result of stimulation of skin-associated lymphoid tissue (SALT).

Steroids, either topically or by injection, rarely affect an established lymphocytoma cutis. The disease is exquisitely radio-sensitive and 300 cGy x 5 at 100 kV will cause complete resolution of the lesions treated with no post-radiotherapy sequelae and no recurrence within the treated field. Occasionally, further patches of lymphocytoma cutis occur outside the treated area and these may be treated similarly. It is assumed therefore that the process had already extended subclinically beyond the initial treatment area prior to the radiotherapy treatment. Some cases of lymphocytoma cutis that have progressed to develop a lymphoma have been described, although this is extremely rare.

LYMPHOMATOID PAPULOSIS

Recurring crops of nodules on the arms and trunk, which ulcerate and then heal leaving scars, characterizes lymphomatoid papulosis[35]. It is of unknown aetiology, affecting both sexes. The lesions are usually small and are often painful before healing. The characteristic scars and the history of spontaneous resolution help with diagnosis. There is generally no lymphadenopathy. Histologically, an infiltrate of extremely atypical lymphoid cells, some of which may be similar to the Sézary cells is seen throughout the dermis. Aggressive histology is at variance with the usually benign nature of the disease. When treatment is necessary, the condition responds to ultraviolet light (UVB) treatment. This disease can sometimes be confused with mycosis fungoides and in some patients mycosis fungoides may co-exist or supervene.

ACKNOWLEDGEMENT

I would like to thank Dr. N. Smith for his help, the Photographic Department at St. John's for the illustrations and above all Miss Elizabeth Pratt for secretarial assistance.

References

1. Edelson, R.L. (1980). Cutaneous T cell lymphoma: Mycosis fungoides, Sézary syndrome and other variants. *J. Am. Acad. Dermatol.*, **2**, 89
2. Wood, G.S. (1983). The immunologic and clinicopathologic heterogeneity of cutaneous lymphomas other than mycosis fungoides. *Blood*, **62**, 464
3. Spittle, M.F. (1977). Mycosis fungoides: electron beam therapy. *Bull. Cancer (Paris)*, **64**, 305
4. Alibert, J.L.M. (1806). *Descriptions des Maladies de la Peau: Observées a l'Hôpital St Louis et Exposition des Meilleures Methodes Suivies pour leur Traitement.* (Paris: Barrois l'Aine et Fils), p.157
5. Bazin, E. (1870). *Leçons sur le Traitement des Maladies Chroniques en Generales Affections de la Peau en Particulier par l'Emploi comparé des Eaux minerales de l'Hydrotherapie et des Moyens Pharmaceutiques* p.425. (Paris: Adrien Delahaye)
6. Vidal, E and Brocq, L. (1885). Étude sur 6 mycosis fungoide. *Fr. Medical* **21**, 946
7. Besnier, E. and Hallopeau, H. (1892). On the erythroderma of mycosis fungoides. *J. Cutan. GenitoUrin. Dis.* **10**, 453
8. Worringer, F. and Kolopp, P. (1939). Lesion erythemato-squameuse polycyclique de l'avant bras évoluant depuis 6 ans chez un garconnet de 13 ans. *Ann. dermatologie venerologie*, **7**, 945
9. Sézary, A. and Bouvrain, Y. (1938). Erythrodermie avec presence de cellules monstreuses dans le derme et le sang circulant. *Bull. Soc. Fr. Dermatol. Syph.*, **45**, 254
10. Lutzner, M.A. and Jordan, J.W. (1968). The ultrastructure of an abnormal cell in Sézary syndrome. *Blood*, **31**, 719
11. Bunn, Jr, P.A. and Lambery, S.I. (1979). Report of the committee on staging and classification of cutaneous T cell lymphomas. *Cancer Treat. Rep.* **63**, 725
12. Cohen, S.R. (1980). Mycosis fungoides: clinicopathologie relationships, sur-

vival and therapy in 59 patients with observations on occupation as a new prognostic factor. *Cancer* **46**, 2654

13. Norris, D.A. and LeFeber, W.P. (1939). Mycosis fungoides and the Sézary. Thiers, B.H. and Dobson, R.L. (eds.). *Pathogenesis of skin disease*. (New York: Churchill Livingstone)
14. Grossman, B., Schechter, G.P., Horton, J.E., *et al.* (1981). A proposal for smoldering adult T cell lymphoma-leukemia. *Am. J. Clin. Pathol.*, **75**, 149
15. Berger, C.L., Rehle, T., Friedman-Kien, A.E., *et al.* (1984). Common membrane antigen on lymphocytes from cutaneous T-cell lymphoma and acquired immune deficiency syndrome patients (Abs). *Clin. Res*, **32**, 571A
16. Robert-Guroff, M. and Gallo, R.C. (1983). Establishment of an etiologic relationship between the human T cell leukemia lymphoma virus (HTLV) and adult T cell leukemia. *Blut*, **47**, 5
17. Castellino, R. and Hoppe, R.T. (1979). Experience with lymphography in patients with mycosis fungoides. *Cancer Treat. Rep.*, **63**, 581
18. Fuks, Z. and Bagshaw, M.A. (1973). Prognostic signs and the management of mycosis fungoides. *Cancer*, **32**, 1385
19. Gilchrest, B.A. and Parrish, J.A. (1976). Oral Methoxsalen photochemotherapy of mycosis fungoides. *Cancer*, **38**, 683
20. Logan, R.A., Spittle, M.F. and Smith, N.P. (1986). Photochemotherapy for cutaneous T-cell lymphomas - the St John's experience. *Br. J. Derm.*, **115**, Suppl. 30, 17
21. Bratherton, D.G. (1972). Strontium beam therapy. In Deeley, T.J. (ed.) *Modern Trends in Radiotherapy*. (London: Butterworths)
22. Vonderheid, E.C. and Van Scott, E.J. (1979). A 10 year experience with topical mechlorethamine for mycosis fungoides: comparison with patients treated by total-skin electron beam radiation therapy. *Cancer Treat. Rep.* **63**, 681
23. Hoppe, R.T., Cox, R.S., Fuks, Z., *et al.* (1979). Electron beam therapy for mycosis fungoides: the Stanford University experience. *Cancer Treat. Rep.* **63**, 691
24. Hoppe, R.T., Fuks, Z. and Bagshaw, M.A. (1977). The rationale for curative radiotherapy in mycosis fungoides. *Int. J. Radiat. Oncol.*, **2**, 843
25. Grozea, P.N. and Jones, S.E. (1979). Combination chemotherapy for mycosis fungoides: A Southwest Oncology Group study. *Cancer Treat. Rep.* **63**, 647
26. Edelson, R.L., Berger, C., Gasparro, F., *et al.* (1983). Treatment of leukemic cutaneous T cell lymphoma with extracorporeally photoactivated 8-methoxypsoralen (abs). *Clin. Res.*, **31**, 467A
27. Braun-Falco, O., Burg, G. and Schmoeckel, C.H. (1981). Recent advances in the understanding of cutaneous lymphoma. *Clin. Exp. Dermatol.* **6**, 89
28. Rappaport, H. (1966). Tumors of the hematopoietic system. In *Atlas of Tumour Pathology*, **3**, 8. (Washington DC: US Armed Forces Institute of Pathology)
29. Lukes, R.J. and Collins, R.D. (1974). Immunological characterization of human malignant lymphomas. *Cancer*, **34**, 1488
30. Lennert, K. and Mori, N. (1974). The histopathology of malignant lymphomas. *Cancer*, **34**, 1488
31. Bennett, M.H., Farrer-Brown, G. and Henry, K. (1974). Classification of non-Hodgkin's lymphomas. *Lancet*, **2**, 405
32. Coltman, Jnr, C.A. *et al.* (1977). Chemotherapy of non-Hodgkin's lymphoma:

10 years' experience in the Southwest Oncology Group. *Cancer Treat. Rep.* **61**, 1067
33. Miller, R.A., Maloney, D.G. and Warnke, R. (1982). Treatment of B cell lymphoma with monoclonal anti-idiotype antibody. *N. Engl. J. Med.* **306**, 577
34. Burg, G. and Braun-Falco, O. (1983). *Cutaneous lymphomas. Pseudolymphomas and related disorders.* (Berlin: Springer-Verlag)
35. Weinman, V.F. and Ackerman, A.B. (1981). Lymphomatoid papulosis: A critical review and new findings. *Am. J. Dermatol.* **3**, 129

4

THE DIAGNOSIS AND MANAGEMENT OF NECROBIOTIC XANTHOGRANULOMA

M. C. FINAN AND R. K. WINKELMANN

INTRODUCTION

Many inflammatory cutaneous diseases and syndromes have been reported to have important or intriguing associations with paraproteinaemia and myeloma. In some of these, the recognition of the cutaneous disease may, through screening laboratory studies, facilitate the diagnosis of an underlying haematological process that may have otherwise escaped clinical notice. While such associations are of interest and of some importance, the pathogenetic relationship between the cutaneous and the haematological processes remains unclear in the vast majority of cases. A list of several such associations is included in Table 4.1. With time, other cutaneous disease processes probably will be added to this list.

This chapter focusses on one specific disease represented in this group – necrobiotic xanthogranuloma – and describes in detail the clinical, pathological, and therapeutic aspects.

OVERVIEW

Necrobiotic xanthogranuloma is a rare clinicopathological entity that is associated with at least one form of paraproteinaemia in most cases reported to date. It is a recently recognized disease process with distinctive features, initially described by Kossard and Winkelmann[1,2] in

TABLE 4.1 Cutaneous diseases associated with myeloma or paraproteinaemia

Amyloidosis
Angioimmunoblastic lymphadenopathy (AILD)
Benign hypergammaglobulinaemia purpura of Waldenström
Dermatitis herpetiformis
Erythema elevatum diutinum
Extramedullary plasmacytoma
Generalized plane xanthomatosis
Necrobiotic xanthogranuloma
POEMS syndrome
Pyoderma gangrenosum
Scleroedema adultorum
Scleromyxoedema
Subcorneal pustular dermatosis

1980. In their review, they described eight patients who had cutaneous lesions of indurated nodules and plaques with a xanthomatous hive. The lesions are distinctive in their tendency to ulcerate, scar, and at times behave aggressively. The histopathological appearance is characterized by a granulomatous infiltrate extending deeply into the dermis and subcutaneous tissue, with xanthomatosis, panniculitis and broad bands of hyaline necrobiosis. Other features found in some of the cases include leukopenia, complement deficiency and bone marrow plasmacytosis, in addition to the more consistent finding of a serum protein abnormality.

Subsequent to the initial series, single and multiple case reports have appeared in the literature. Holden *et al.*[3] reported four cases, Codère *et al.*[4] reported two cases, and additional single cases have been published by Macfarlane and Verbov[5], Smith *et al.*[6], Kocsard[7], Marchat[8], and Hunter and Burry[9]. The ophthalmological findings in 16 cases of necrobiotic xanthogranuloma were reviewed by Robertson and Winkelmann[10]. The cases in the last study, as well as those reported in the initial series of Kossard and Winkelmann, were included in the review by Finan and Winkelmann[11], which describes the clinical and pathological findings in 22 cases of necrobiotic xanthogranuloma. The details of the histopathological findings in these 22 cases have been published elsewhere[12].

Necrobiotic xanthogranuloma has been reported as atypical necrobiosis lipoidica[13,14], atypical multicentric reticulohistiocytosis with paraproteinaemia[15], lymphocytoma developing into xanthogranuloma[16], and as unusual forms of xanthoma disseminatum[17-19], among others.

The material that follows describes, in detail, the clinical and histopathological findings, the diagnosis and differential diagnosis, and the management of necrobiotic xanthogranuloma. Most of the data have been derived from the series reported by Finan and Winkelmann[11,12].

CLINICAL FINDINGS

Clinically, the cutaneous lesions of necrobiotic xanthogranuloma are seen as indurated papules, nodules, or plaques, which are red-orange to violaceous and often display a yellowish or xanthomatous hive. Secondary changes of scarring, telangiectasia and atrophy are observed frequently; in addition, surface ulcers have been noted. Ten of the 22 patients described by Finan and Winkelmann had surface lesions, some of which were extensive (Figure 4.1). The sizes of the lesions vary greatly from a few millimetres to several centimetres in diameter. Some lesions have evolved from small papules to large plaques with central depression. The lesions were asymptomatic in 13 of the 22 patients. However, six patients complained of lesional pain or tenderness (or both), four complained of pruritus, and two described a burning discomfort.

Lesions most characteristically involved the periorbital area (21 of 22 patients), as is commonly found in other xanthomatoses. The trunk, extremities, and other areas of the face were also frequent sites of involvement. Multiple lesions were seen in all 22 patients, and frequently the lesions were bilateral and symmetrical.

Periorbital lesions tended to be more aggressive and disfiguring than lesions at other sites. In two patients, the lesions progressed to complete blindness secondary to orbital destruction by necrobiotic xanthogranuloma. Ophthalmic symptoms and findings were frequent. Painful, itchy or burning eyes (or combinations of these) were described by 7 of the 22 patients. Changes in visual acuity, including blurred or hazy vision, diplopia, or acute transient visual loss, were described by seven patients. Inflammatory changes of episcleritis,

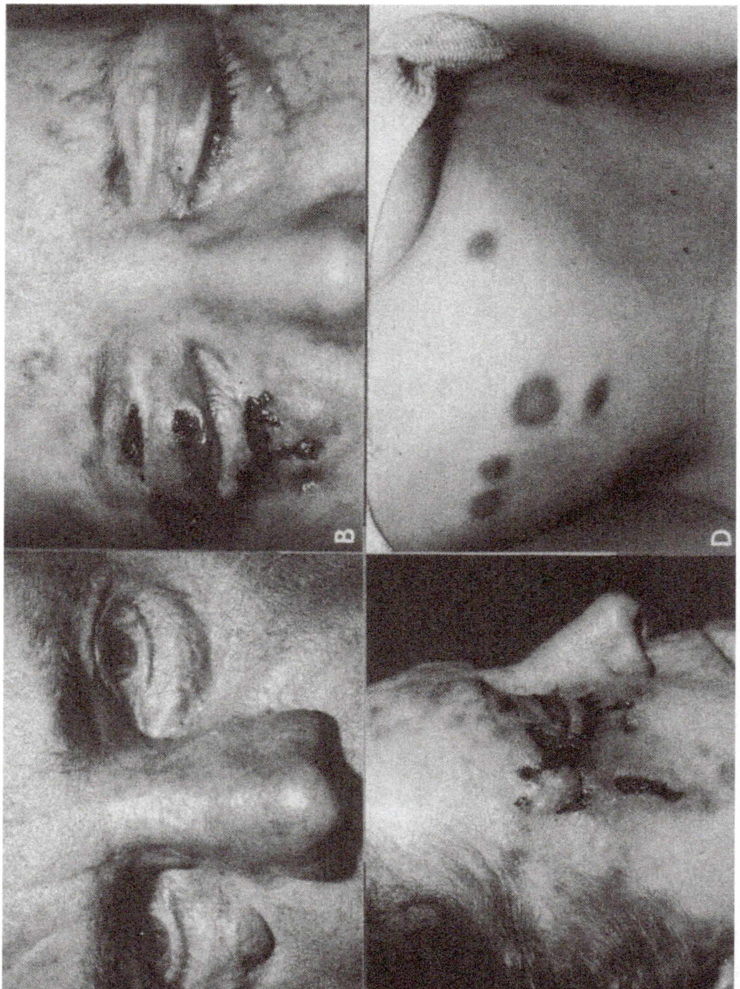
A
B
C
D

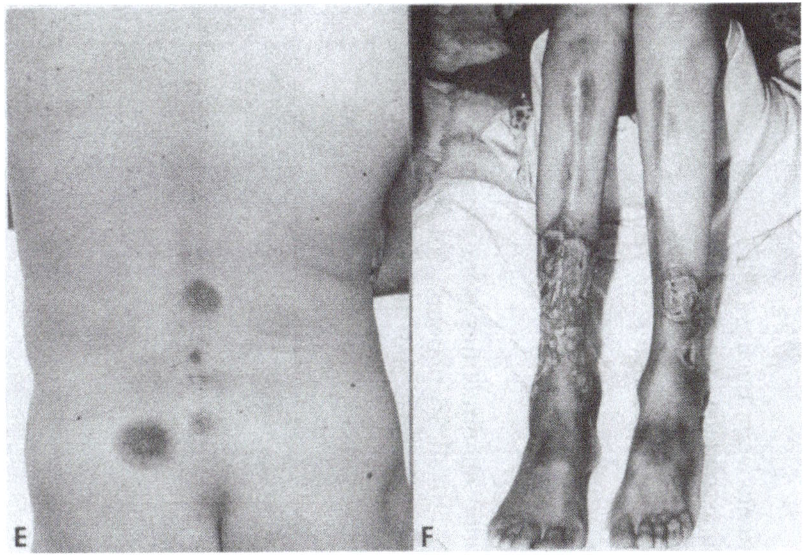

FIGURE 4.1 Necrobiotic xanthogranuloma. (A) Early lesions, simulating xanthelasma; (B) later lesions, showing induration and ulceration of periorbital tissue; (C) lateral view, showing destructive ulceration in periorbital necrobiotic xanthogranuloma; (D) and (E) indurated, annular plaques on trunk; (F) ulcerative lesion involving lower extremities (and other areas not shown), simulating necrobiosis lipoidica. [(B) From Robertson and Winkelmann[10]. Published with permission from the American Journal of Ophthalmology. Copyright The Ophthalmic Publishing Company. (C) and (D) From Kossard and Winkelmann[2]. By permission of the American Academy of Dermatology. (E) from Winkelmann and Welborn[16]. By permission of Springer-Verlag]

scleritis, uveitis and iritis were found in some patients, and ptosis and glaucoma occasionally affected patients. Two patients complained of dry eyes, but a sicca syndrome was not documented. Rare findings included proptosis secondary to orbital tumour, exophthalmos, ectropion, exposure keratitis, and ocular myalgia.

None of the 22 patients with necrobiotic xanthogranuloma had lymphadenopathy. Hepatomegaly, splenomegaly, or both were documented in six patients. Five patients had arthritis or arthralgias (or both).

Thirteen of the 22 patients were females (M:F, 1:1.4). Twenty-one of the 22 patients had an associated systemic disease. The mean age of these 21 at onset of the cutaneous disease and at diagnosis of the systemic abnormality was the same, that is, 53 years.

LABORATORY FINDINGS

One or more serum protein abnormalities were present in 20 of the 22 patients (Table 4.2). In all 16 patients with monoclonal gammopathy, the paraprotein was IgG, and the light-chain component

TABLE 4.2 Types of paraproteinaemia in 22 patients with necrobiotic xanthogranuloma[a]

	Patients	
Type	*No.*	*%*
Monoclonal gammopathy	16	73.0
Alone	11	
With multiple myeloma	2	
With cryoglobulinaemia	2	
With chronic lymphocytic leukaemia	1	
Cryoglobulinaemia	2	9.0
Multiple myeloma	1	4.5
Abnormal serum protein electrophoresis[b]	1	4.5
No paraproteinaemia	2	9.0
Total	**22**	**100.0**

a From Finan and Winkelmann[11]. By permission of the Williams & Wilkins Company

b Immunoelectrophoresis not done

was of both κ (8 patients) and λ (7 patients) subtypes; typing was not done in one patient. Other significant paraprotein findings included cryoglobulinaemia in four patients, multiple myeloma in three, and an abnormal serum protein electrophoresis, which was not further evaluated, in one patient. Of the two remaining patients without paraproteinaemia, one had a mild elevation of serum triglyceride level and the second had mild diabetes mellitus and an abnormal lipoprotein electrophoregram. In general, however, serum protein abnormalities seemed to be a consistent finding in patients with necrobiotic xanthogranuloma.

Other laboratory abnormalities were common with necrobiotic xanthogranuloma. These included elevation of the erythrocyte sedimentation rate, leukopenia, complement deficiency and anaemia (Table 4.3). A positive antinuclear antibody, rheumatoid factor, and thrombocytopenia were infrequent findings. Three patients had an elevated fasting blood glucose level on at least one occasion, but the elevations were modest, and none of the patients was insulin-dependent. Microscopic haematuria, without evidence of urinary tract

TABLE 4.3 Laboratory abnormalities in 22 patients with necrobiotic xanthogranuloma[a]

	Patients	
Finding	*Tested*	*With abnormal results*
Increased erythrocyte sedimentation rate	22	20
Leukopenia	22	13
Absolute neutropenia	22	10
Decreased CH_{50}	14	7
Decreased C4	11	6
Decreased C1-esterase inhibitor	3	2
Serum protein abnormality	22	20
Bone marrow examination		
Plasmacytosis/plasmaproliferative disorder	17	7
Myeloma	17	3
Lymphoproliferative disorder	17	2
Non-diagnostic	17	5

a From Finan and Winkelmann[11]. By permission of the Williams & Wilkins Company

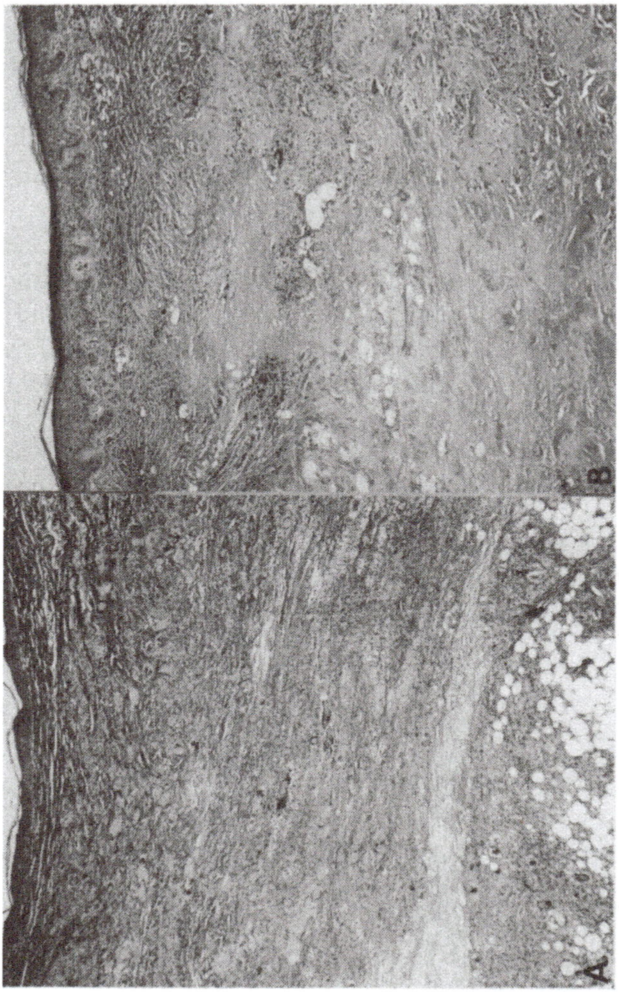
A
B

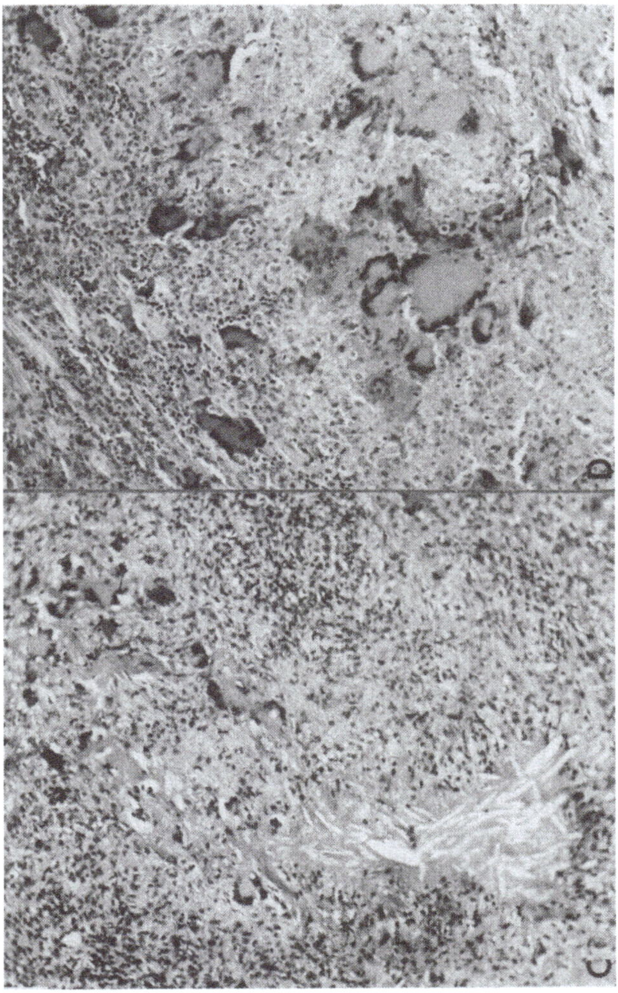

FIGURE 4.2 (A) Lesion showing granulomatous infiltrate throughout dermis, with extension into panniculus (Haematoxylin and eosin, x 40); (B) Lesion showing broad zones of hyaline necrobiosis within background of giant cells and granulomatous inflammation (haematoxylin and eosin, x 64); (C) higher power showing granulomatous infiltrate with cholesterol clefts and numerous giant cells of somewhat unusual appearance (haematoxylin and eosin, x 160); (D) higher power showing numerous giant cells embedded in granulomatous inflammation (haematoxylin and eosin, x 160)

infection, was found in five patients; delayed hypersensitivity skin testing in four patients showed anergy in only one patient. Serum triglyceride, cholesterol or total lipid levels were measured in all but three patients. Four patients had hypertriglyceridaemia, and two had hypercholesterolaemia, but elevations were mild in most patients. One of these patients had type IIa familial hypercholesterolaemia. Bone marrow aspirate and biopsy were performed in 17 patients. Plasmacytosis was found in seven, sometimes in association with atypical plasma cells; overt myeloma was found in three; and lymphocytosis was present in two (one of whom had known chronic lymphocytic leukemia). In five other patients, the study was non-diagnostic. Bone scans or surveys (or both), as well as roentgenograms of the orbit, were normal in all patients tested.

Extracutaneous granulomatous disease was documented in only one case of our series, with evidence of pulmonary involvement. We are aware of one other case in the literature with visceral xanthogranulomas – that of Hunter and Burry [9] – with lesions in the kidney, larynx and heart as well as the skin. As this entity becomes more widely recognized, and as more autopsy cases are examined, perhaps the incidence of extracutaneous involvement will be seen to be significantly more prevalent than suggested by the data currently available.

HISTOPATHOLOGICAL FINDINGS

The salient histopathological findings in cutaneous necrobiotic xanthogranuloma include (1) a granulomatous dermal or subcutaneous (or both) inflammatory infiltrate (Figure 4.2A), sometimes with Touton cell panniculitis; (2) xanthomatization of histiocytes and giant cells; (3) the striking presence of giant cells of both the Touton cell and foreign-body types, the latter often being unusual in appearance; (4) the presence of broad bands of hyaline necrobiosis (Figure 4.2B); and (5) the variable, but characteristic, presence of cholesterol clefts (Figure 4.2C), lymphoid nodules, and foci of plasma cells.

Granulomatous masses, consisting of histiocytes, giant cells, and lesser numbers of lymphocytes, are found within (and often replace) large portions of the dermis or subcutaneous tissue (or both). Broad bands of hyaline necrobiosis impart a somewhat lobulated appearance to the tissue. Numerous Touton giant cells, as well as foreign-body giant cells of rather bizarre appearance, may be present, often near areas of hyaline necrobiosis. The foreign-body giant cells are unusual in their frequently irregular shape, size, and arrangement of nuclei (Figure 4.2D). Although Touton cell panniculitis is a distinctive feature of necrobiotic xanthogranuloma, it is not always present.

Diagnostically helpful features that may be present include cholesterol clefts, lymphoid nodules (Figure 4.3), and foci of plasma cells.

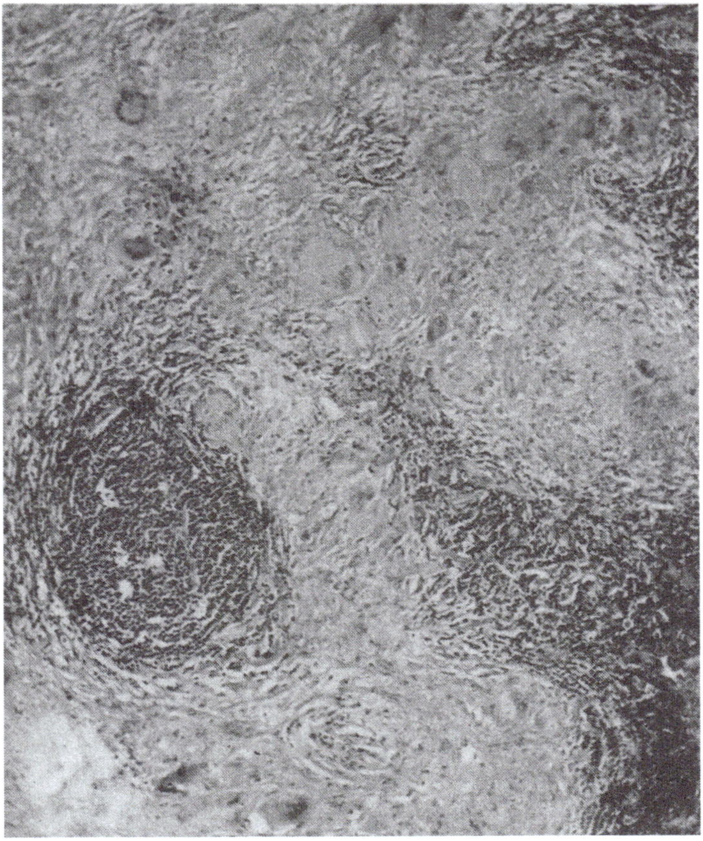

FIGURE 4.3 Lymphoid nodule and lymphocytic inflammation within background of granulomatous inflammation with numerous giant cells of both the Touton and foreign-body types (haematoxylin and eosin, x 100)

Cholesterol clefts are seen as slit-like clear spaces within the dermis and subcutaneous tissue, usually within areas of necrobiosis. Lymphoid nodules are found, most often in the lower part of the dermis, and nodules with germinal centre formation may simulate lymphocytoma. Plasma cells most often have a perivascular distribution, but they also are found at the periphery of lymphoid nodules. The granulomatous infiltrate tends to extend deeply into the subcutaneous tissue, and infiltration between muscle bundles is an occasional finding. An interesting and unique observation in two specimens was a 'palisading cholesterol cleft granuloma' in the dermis, consisting of a peripheral palisade of foamy histiocytes with central cholesterol clefting. Granules that are periodic-acid–Schiff positive and diastase resistant are found, often in a ring-like pattern, within the giant cells and histiocytes.

Direct immunofluorescence study of cutaneous lesions (11 specimens) yielded variable results, the most frequent finding being fluorescence of the deep cutaneous vasculature with IgM, C3, or fibrin (or combinations of these).

Leukocyte monoclonal antibody studies from involved skin of six patients showed an infiltrate staining primarily with OKM1, or cells of the monocyte-macrophage series. Helper-inducer T cells (OKT4, Leu-3a) were also present in the infiltrate, and significant numbers of suppressor/cytotoxic T cells (OKT8, Leu-2a) were observed.

Three specimens failed to show significant anti-S100 protein reactivity in histiocytes and giant cells, as previously reported[20].

DIAGNOSIS AND DIFFERENTIAL DIAGNOSIS

The diagnosis of necrobiotic xanthogranuloma should be made by correlation of clinical findings with its rather distinctive histopathological pattern. Various xanthomatous and granulomatous processes may be considered in the differential diagnosis, from both a clinical and histological standpoint. Included most often in the clinical differential diagnosis are xanthelasma, necrobiosis lipoidica, juvenile xanthogranuloma, generalized plane normolipaemic xanthoma, xanthoma disseminatum, and the various xanthomas associated with hyperlipidaemia. Of this group, xanthelasma and necrobiosis lipoidica are most frequently confused with necrobiotic xanthogranuloma clinically. Periorbital lesions, found almost universally in necrobiotic xanthogranuloma, may prompt an initial diagnosis of xanthelasma. However, the tendency to aggressive ulceration and scarring in necrobiotic xanthogranuloma, in addition to the induration of individual lesions, the frequent presence of lesions elsewhere on the body and a histopathological pattern that is different from the pattern of xanthelasma, should lead to the correct diagnosis. Individual lesions of necrobiosis lipoidica may closely resemble lesions of necrobiotic xanthogranuloma, particularly when the latter lesions are located in a pretibial distribution. Five of the 22 patients in our series had pretibial lesions, but again, the presence of ulcers and paraprotein abnormalities and the lack of diabetes mellitus, along with the histopathological findings of necrobiotic xanthogranuloma, should aid in the differentiation.

Necrobiosis lipoidica, granuloma annulare, juvenile xanthogranuloma, Rothmann–Makai panniculitis, erythema induratum, foreign-body granuloma, atypical sarcoid, and the various xanthomas may be included in the histological differential diagnosis of necrobiotic xanthogranuloma. Of these, necrobiosis lipoidica is the most difficult to differentiate from necrobiotic xanthogranuloma. The granulomatous infiltrate of necrobiotic xanthogranuloma tends to be more cellular, and the giant cells are more prominent and atypical than is classically seen in necrobiosis lipoidica. In necrobiotic xanthogranuloma, lipid deposition tends to be more limited in extent, with Oil Red O stain showing only focal lipid droplets within the giant cells and areas of necrobiosis. Lymphoid nodules have not, to our knowledge, been described in necrobiosis lipoidica, and cholesterol clefts are rare.

While the presence of a serum protein abnormality may lend support to a diagnosis of necrobiotic xanthogranuloma in patients with the appropriate clinical and histopathological features, its presence is not mandatory for the diagnosis. As noted previously, 2 of our 22 patients lacked paraproteinaemia despite a characteristic clinicopathological pattern. Also, the possibility remains that a paraproteinaemia will develop subsequent to the clinical/cutaneous presentation.

In patients in whom the diagnosis of necrobiotic xanthogranuloma is seriously considered, we recommend examining skin biopsy specimens and doing a thorough laboratory evaluation. Studies should include a complete chemistry profile, complete blood count with differential count, erythrocyte sedimentation rate, serum lipid profile, bone marrow aspirate and biopsy, chest roentgenogram, urinalysis, roentgenograms of long bones and the orbit and serum complement studies (CH_{50}, C3, C4 and C1 esterase inhibitor). Immunophoretic studies may be performed, pending results of a screening protein electrophoresis.

COURSE AND MANAGEMENT

In general, the course of the cutaneous disease in necrobiotic xanthogranuloma is slowly progressive, with a gradual enlargement of pre-existing lesions and the development of new lesions over time. Occasionally, a few lesions may resolve spontaneously, similar to the case in other cutaneous non-X histiocytoses. When present, the myeloma process in necrobiotic xanthogranuloma tends to be significantly more prolonged in course and benign in nature than the usual, more fulminant, type of myeloma. Destructive bony lesions and Bence Jones proteinuria are rare.

A number of therapeutic modalities were employed in our series of patients with necrobiotic xanthogranuloma, in the treatment of both the cutaneous and the systemic disease. Chemotherapeutic agents, alone or in conjunction with systemic steroids, were given to 18 patients. Specifically, these agents were chlorambucil alone (six patients), melphalan alone (three patients), melphalan with prednisone (two patients), cyclophosphamide alone (two patients), azathioprine alone (two patients), chlorambucil with prednisone (one patient), nitrogen mustard (one patient), and methotrexate (one patient). The response to therapy was somewhat difficult to assess, both because of the wide variety of agents employed and the inconsistent follow-up. Transient improvement or partial remissions were noted in the group as a whole, but recurrences were common. Improvement was most notable, however, in patients given low-dose chlorambucil, with shrinkage in lesion size or disappearance of pre-existing lesions (or both).

Response to local therapy, such as surgical excision and intralesional or topically applied steroids, was generally poor. Local radiation therapy to the involved skin in one patient, however, led to a significant shrinkage in lesion size, and this may represent a viable therapeutic option in selected patients.

On the basis of this somewhat limited experience, our current choice of therapy for patients with unifocal cutaneous disease is X-ray treatment. For more extensive involvement, the use of a low-dose alkylating agent – specifically, chlorambucil in a dose of 2–4 mg by mouth daily – is suggested. Low-dose therapy is preferred because a significant number of patients with necrobiotic xanthogranuloma have a pre-existing leukopenia. The physician may elect to add prednisone to the chlorambucil therapy, depending on the nature of the underlying disease, the degree of inflammation present in existing lesions, and individual preference. Further experience is needed in this area to better define optimal therapeutic regimens.

REFERENCES

1. Kossard, S. and Winkelmann, R.K. (1980). Necrobiotic xanthogranuloma. *Australas. J. Dermatol.*, **21,** 85–8
2. Kossard, S. and Winkelmann, R.K. (1980). Necrobiotic xanthogranuloma with paraproteinemia. *J. Am. Acad. Dermatol.*, **3,** 257–70
3. Holden, C.A., Winkelmann, R.K. and Wilson Jones, E. (1986). Necrobiotic xanthogranuloma: a report of four cases. *Br. J. Dermatol.*, **114,** 241–50
4. Codère, F., Lee, R.D. and Anderson, R.L. (1983). Necrobiotic xanthogranuloma of the eyelid. *Arch. Ophthalmol.*,**101,** 60–3
5. Macfarlane, A.W. and Verbov, J.L. (1985). Necrobiotic xanthogranuloma with paraproteinaemia. *Br. J. Dermatol.*, **113,** 339–43
6. Smith, S.A., Alexander, R.A., Stasko, T., Roberts, L.C. and Stevens, C.S. (1983). Necrobiotic xanthogranuloma. *J. Assoc. Milit. Dermatol.*, **9,** 78–80
7. Kocsard, E. (1983). Xantogranuloma necrobiotico con paraproteinemia. *G. Ital. Dermatol. Venereol.*, **118,** 219–22
8. Marchat, C. (1985). Xanthogranulome necrobiotique est dysglobulineme monoclonale: a propos d'une observation. These pour le doctorate en medicine, Universite Pierre et Marie Curie, Faculté de Medecine Saint-Antoine, Paris.
9. Hunter, L. and Burry, A.F. (1985). Necrobiotic xanthogranuloma: a systemic disease with paraproteinemia. *Pathology.* **17,** 533-6
10. Robertson, D.M. and Winkelmann, R.K. (1984). Ophthalmic features of necrobiotic xanthogranuloma with paraproteinemia. *Am. J. Ophthalmol.* **97,** 173–83
11. Finan, M.C. and Winkelmann, R.K. (1986). Necrobiotic xanthogranuloma with paraproteinemia: a review of 22 cases. *Medicine (Baltimore)*, **65,** 376–88
12. Finan, M.C. and Winkelmann, R.K. (1987). Histopathology of necrobiotic xanthogranuloma with paraproteinemia. *J. Cutan. Pathol.*, **14,** 92–99

13. Muller, S.A. and Winkelmann, R.K. (1966). Atypical forms of necrobiosis lipoidica diabeticorum: a report of three cases. *Arch. Pathol.* **81,** 352–61
14. Wantzin, G.L., Siim, E. and Medgyesi, S. (1980). An unusual example of necrobiosis lipoidica affecting the face. *Br. J. Plast. Surg.,* **33,** 61–3
15. Rendall, J.R.S., Vanhegan, R.I., Robb-Smith, A.H.T., Bowers, R.E., Ryan, T.J. and Vickers, H.R. (1977). Atypical multicentric reticulohistiocytosis with paraproteinemia. *Arch. Dermatol.,* **113,** 1576–82
16. Winkelmann, R.K. and Welborn, W.R. (1969). Xanthome und maligne retikulosen. *Hautarzt,* **20,** 550–5
17. Frank, S.B. (1977). Xanthomatous granuloma. *Arch. Dermatol.,* **113,** 1450
18. Frank, S.B. and Weidman, A.I. (1952). Xanthoma disseminatum: an unusual form with extension of xanthomatous changes into muscle. *Arch. Dermatol. Syph.* **65,** 88–94
19. Maize, J.C., Ahmed, A.R. and Provost, T.T. (1974). Xanthoma disseminatum and multiple myeloma. *Arch. Dermatol.,* **110,** 758–61
20. Winkelmann, R.K., Venencie, P.Y., Rowden, G. (1983). S–100 protein identification of Langerhans' cells and histiocytosis X cutaneous disease (abstract). *Arch. Dermatol.,* **119,** 847–8

5

THE DIAGNOSIS AND MANAGEMENT OF SCLEROMYXOEDEMA

A. W. MACFARLANE AND J. L. VERBOV

Scleromyxoedema is a variant of lichen myxoedematosus (papular mucinosis), one of the primary cutaneous mucinoses. The disease is rare and the aetiology is unknown. The characteristic features are (1) infiltrative skin lesions due to deposition of acid mucopolysaccharide in the dermis; (2) normal thyroid function; and (3) a serum paraprotein which is found in most, but not all, cases[1]. The clinical and histological appearances, paraproteinaemia, complications, and management will be discussed.

CLINICAL APPEARANCE

A number of distinct clinical types of lichen myxoedematosus have been documented since the original description of the disease by Dubreuilh[2] in 1906. The four variants described by Montgomery and Underwood[3] in 1953 were (1) a generalized lichenoid eruption with discrete papules over the entire body, especially affecting the hands, forearms, face, neck and the upper part of the trunk; (2) a discrete papular eruption on the trunk and extremities; (3) localized or generalized lichenoid papules over the body; and (4) urticarial plaques and nodular eruptions. In 1954, Gottron[4] credited Arndt with the term 'scleromyxoedema' to describe the generalized form of the disease; some later reports use this term synonymously with lichen myxoedematosus. A form has also been described in which there are nodulocystic lesions[5,6].

The condition is not confined to Caucasian skin: its occurrence in Negroes, for example, is well documented[3,7–13]. The literature reveals a slight preponderance of male cases, and the incidence is highest in the fourth to seventh decades.

Clinically, scleromyxoedema is characterized by diffuse skin involvement and the appearance of uniform, flesh-coloured, dome-shaped papules on skin that is erythematous, infiltrated and palpably thickened owing to deposition of acid mucopolysaccharide in the dermis[14]. The diameter of the papules ranges from pinhead-size to about 3mm[3,8,14].

The arms, chest and face (especially the glabellar area) are often the worst-affected areas[1,5,8,13,15–17], the skin infiltration leading to thickened furrows on the face and a coarse appearance that has been described as wax-like[18,19]. Facial expression and jaw movement may be so severely limited that wearing or removal of dentures, or even eating, become impossible[1,3,5,6,8,9,14,16–21], and infiltration of the digital skin may impair walking or result in an inability to flex or extend the fingers fully[8,9,17,19]. The skin overlying joints is thrown into rugose folds, but remains mobile (Figures 5.1 and 5.2). Pruritus may be troublesome[5,8,12,13,22,23]. The condition is slowly progressive.

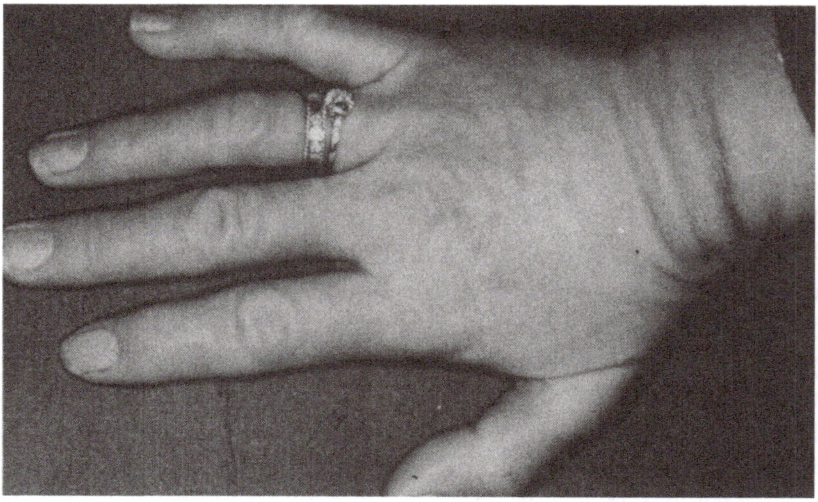

FIGURE 5.1 Thickened skin folds over wrist due to infiltration of dermis with acid mucopolysaccharide

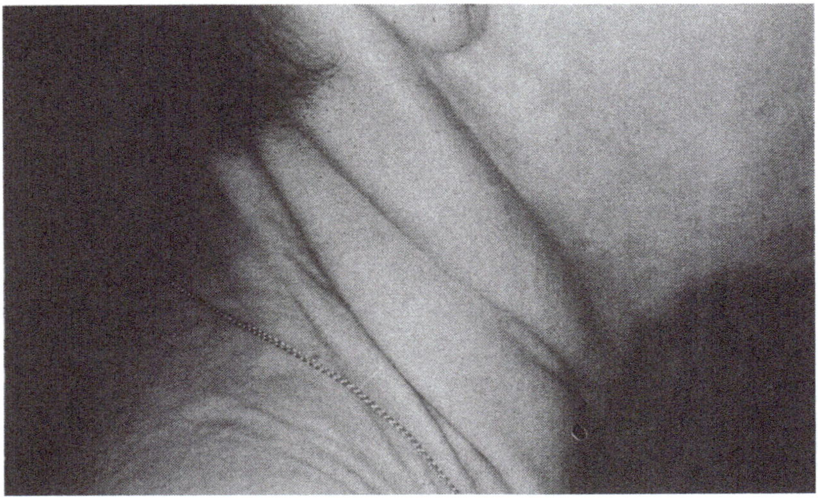

FIGURE 5.2 Grossly thickened folds of skin on neck due to infiltration of dermis with acid mucopolysaccharide

An initial presentation with facial involvement and acrosclerosis may be mistaken for scleroderma. However, in scleromyxoedema the skin is not bound down to underlying tissues, unlike the case of scleroderma. There may be clinical and histological similarities with myxoedema, but thyroid function is normal in scleromyxoedema. With very few exceptions, further investigation in scleromyxoedema reveals a serum paraprotein.

HISTOLOGY

Histologically, there is proliferation of abnormal stellate and spindle-shaped fibroblasts, and deposition of acid mucopolysaccharide in the upper part of the dermis (Figures 5.3 and 5.4)[8]. The collagen fibres appear separated into a loose network. The presence of acid mucopolysaccharide may be demonstrated by positive-staining with Alcian blue (usually with a PAS counterstain), colloidal iron, or mucicarmine[7–9,13,14,18,22]; it stains metachromatically with toluidine blue and azure A[7,14,18,24]. The acid mucopolysaccharide consists mainly of

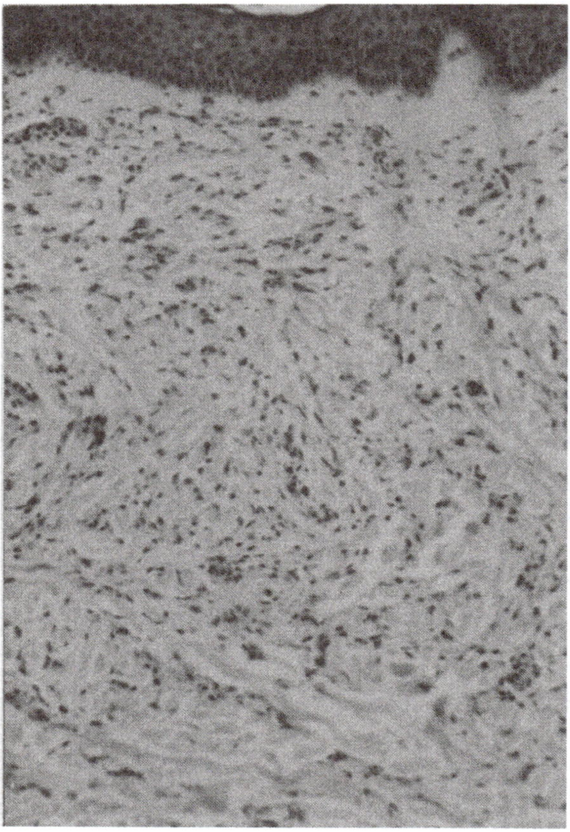

FIGURE 5.3 Irregular collagen bundles and proliferation of fibroblasts in upper dermis (haematoxylin and eosin x 130)

hyaluronic acid and it is largely removed by hyaluronidase[3,5,8,9,14]. Staining for amyloid is negative[14,22].

In some cases, there is a mixed but mainly lymphocytic infiltrate around appendages and blood vessels[7,14,23]. Eosinophils may be seen between fibroblasts[8,12] and mast cells may be increased[14,24,25]. The epidermis appears normal, although there may be thinning and effacement of the rete pegs due to the presence of mucin in the dermis[3,14].

Immunofluorescence of skin produces variable results. In most cases it is negative[1,5,9,16,21,24–29], but some cases have demonstrated immunoglobulin in areas of mucin deposition[18,22,30].

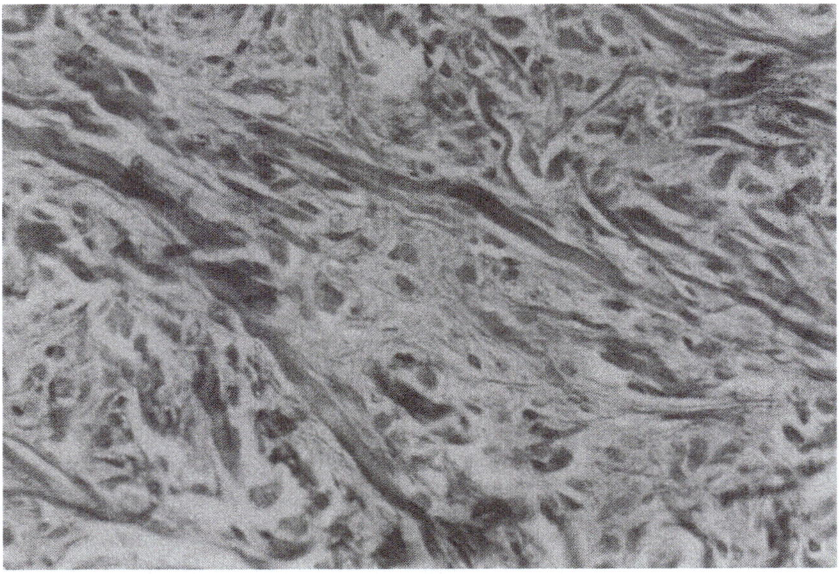

FIGURE 5.4 Irregular collagen bundles separated by acid mucopolysaccharide deposition (Alcian blue, x 300)

PARAPROTEIN

In 1960, Perry, Montgomery and Stickney[14] reported an abnormal serum protein in a patient with lichen myxoedematosus. Abnormal plasma cells were found in the bone marrow, and they considered this to be the first reported case of lichen myxoedematosus occurring in association with multiple myeloma. It was recognized, however, that other cases of lichen myxoedematosus pursued a relatively benign course compared with multiple myeloma (survival was longer, they were not associated with systemic complications such as hypercalcaemia or osteolytic bone lesions, and Bence Jones proteinuria was absent) and in this case it was acknowledged that the association between the two diseases was likely to be coincidental. (In fact, the original diagnosis of multiple myeloma could not later be substantiated using modern criteria[13].)

It soon became clear, however, that lichen myxoedematosus was indeed associated with the presence of an abnormal, homogeneous, extremely basic (cathodic) serum globulin that migrated in the post-gamma region on electrophoresis[16,18]. This abnormal globulin was recognized to be a myeloma-type protein[18], and later characterized as an IgG paraprotein with λ light chains[9,16,31]. The paraprotein was found to be more basic in nature than myeloma paraproteins generally, a characteristic that is related to the structure of the Fab fragment[16,32]. In a study of five patients, the IgG subtype was IgG_1 in all cases[32].

Since then, nearly all reported cases of scleromyxoedema have been associated with an IgG λ paraproteinaemia. There are also reports of an IgG κ paraprotein[23,24,33], elevation of serum IgA[21], a biclonal paraprotein (IgGλ and IgA λ)[34] and Waldenström's macroglobulinaemia[35]. Hill, Crawford and Rogers suggested that the presence of a paraprotein was a necessary criterion for the diagnosis of lichen myxoedematosus[1], but there are cases in which no paraprotein was found[12,22,36] and in which it could not be demonstrated until several years after the appearance of the skin changes[27]. The relationship between the paraprotein level and the extent of skin involvement is not clear. In one case, the paraprotein persisted for several years after the spontaneous resolution of the skin disease[37], and in another it was found three years before the onset of the skin disease[28]. Successful treatment does not always decrease the level of paraprotein[34].

It has been shown that paraprotein synthesis may take place both in the bone marrow and in the skin[24], and further research into the cutaneous mucinoses has shown that sera from patients with some mucinous conditions (*viz.* scleromyxoedema, pretibial myxoedema or scleroedema) may stimulate fibroblasts in one way or another. Harper and Rispler[11], for example, found that sera from patients with lichen myxoedematosus would stimulate skin fibroblast proliferation *in vitro*. Sera from patients with Graves' disease and pretibial myxoedema was shown by Cheung *et al.*[38] to induce fibroblast cultures to elaborate hyaluronic acid, and, more recently, Ohta *et al.*[39] showed that sera from patients who had paraproteinaemias associated with scleroedema (as distinct from scleromyxoedema) stimulated the production of collagen in fibroblast cultures. The fact that the common features described in these papers are, firstly, an abnormal serum immunoglobulin (long-acting thyroid-stimulating immunoglobulin in the case of Graves' disease) and, secondly, stimulation by serum of fibroblast activity, suggests that the skin changes seen in these conditions somehow result from the stimulation of dermal fibroblasts by the abnormal circulating globulin. Tempting though it is to speculate on these lines, however, current experimental and clinical evidence indicates that the immunoglobulin itself is *not* the agent responsible for stimulating fibroblast activity[11,38], and that the serum factor that is actually responsible remains unidentified. Although the abnormal immunoglobulin may be a marker for scleromyxoedema, it does not appear to have an aetiological role[40].

Bone marrow examination in most cases is normal and it follows that lichen myxoedematosus is not generally a skin manifestation of myeloma. However, it is worthwhile noting that some patients have had evidence of plasma cell hyperplasia[14,17,18,29] or actual multiple myeloma[13], and that one case has been described in association with Waldenström's macroglobulinaemia[35]. It is therefore reasonable to recommend bone marrow examination of all patients with scleromyxoedema.

The paraprotein does not seem to be directed against an endogenous antigen (e.g., hyaluronic acid) and the disease cannot, therefore, be considered to be autoimmune in origin[24,32].

COMPLICATIONS AND ASSOCIATED CONDITIONS

Neurological complications

The most frequently reported systemic complications of scleromyxoedema are episodes of neurological dysfunction. They include headache[27], disorientation[25], mental deterioration[7], changes in level of consciousness[24], dysarthria[17,24,27], ataxia[25], limb weakness or paralysis[14,27], hemiparesis[25], fits[24,25] and coma. One patient developed lichen myxoedematosus while convalescing from an unexplained 'encephalitis'[15].

Although in some cases episodes of neurological dysfunction seem to be associated with scleromyxoedema *per se* and are otherwise unexplained, it is clearly important to exclude coexistent neurological disease. Rudner, Mehregan and Pinkus[8] reported two fatal cases with marked neurological dysfunction, including dysarthria, localized and generalized fits, hemiparesis and coma; in the first case an episode of aphasia preceded the development of lichen myxoedematosus[8]. However, post-mortem examination revealed causes for the neurological dysfunction other than lichen myxoedematosus. The first patient was found to have bilateral subdural haematomas and the second to have tuberculous leptomeningitis. Jepsen reported two cases of scleromyxoedema: in one, herpetic encephalitis had preceded the eruption and in the other a meningioma was present[6]. In another fatal case it was felt that vascular occlusive disease was responsible for the neurological symptoms[25].

Post-mortem findings

Widespread mucin deposition is rarely found at post-mortem examination, despite marked systemic symptoms[8,14,24], and its presence in the brain has not been documented. Even the presence of mucin in a number of organs may be the result of local degenerative changes in those organs, rather than an indication of systemic mucin deposition[25].

One of the original patients of Montgomery and Underwood was shown at autopsy to have mucin deposited in the walls of cutaneous blood vessels and nerve bundles, coronary vessels, and the perivascular connective tissue of the kidney, adrenal and pancreas; in addition, there was focal demyelination and gliosis in the central nervous system[7]. The original interpretation of these findings as indicating mucin deposition due to lichen myxoedematosus has been challenged – this patient had also suffered severe weight loss, and had degeneration and lymphocytic infiltration of skeletal muscle and myocardium that was probably secondary to poor nutrition and local damage[25]. Another patient showed mucin deposition in renal papillae[14] but, again, this may have been secondary to inflammation at this site[25].

In addition to the neurological diseases described above, some patients have shown puzzling pathological findings at post-mortem examination. A patient who had had numbness of the extremities, incoordination and later paraplegia was found to have multiple central nervous system infarcts, but no widespread mucin deposition[14]. Another, with severe neurological symptoms, had cerebral oedema at autopsy, but no other relevant abnormality[24].

Proppe *et al.*[41], reported the presence of congophilic material (amyloid) in the skin, many internal organs, and blood vessels in a case of scleromyxoedema, but there are no other reports of systemic amyloid deposition. A fatal case with post-mortem evidence of mucin in the oesophagus and submucosa of the large bowel seems to have had Degos' syndrome (malignant atrophic pustulosis) rather than lichen myxoedematosus[42].

Other associated diseases

Muldrow and Bailin[13] reported a case of multiple myeloma with scleromyxoedema, and quoted four other definite cases. In addition to the disorders mentioned above, other diseases reported in association with scleromyxoedema or lichen myxoedematosus include dermatomyositis[10], pachydermoperiostosis[25], coronary artery disease[8,12,14,18], cerebrovascular accident[12] and ankylosing spondylitis[43]. One patient was felt to have concomitant hypothyroidism and scleroderma with oesophageal aperistalsis[34], although Alligood *et al.*[12] considered oesophageal aperistalsis a complication of scleromyxoedema itself. One patient had a pancreatic tumour and another had a gastric carcinoma, both probably coincidental[25]. A recently described patient had multiple keratoacanthomas[33].

MANAGEMENT

Because of its rarity, reports of the treatment of scleromyxoedema usually deal with only one or two patients. Evidence regarding the success of various treatments must therefore largely be built up from a comparison of individual case reports.

A large number of agents have been tried, many on a purely empirical basis. Most have been found to be ineffective or, at best, of equivocal value. These have included α-tocopherol[1,21], vitamin A[3,12], quinacrine[14], urethane[14], thyroid extract[3,14,18], iodides[3], nitrogen mustard[14,29], intralesional hyaluronidase[3,8], topical hyaluronidase[19], oral oestrogens[3,37], penicillamine[6] and edetic acid (EDTA)[1]. One patient showed some improvement with ACTH[19], but in general there is no response to prednisone alone[3,12,14,18,20,22,28,29,37,42] or to topical steroids[19,23,27,29].

Cytotoxic agents

Melphalan

The first report of the successful use of melphalan in scleromyxoedema came in 1969[31]. An initial loading dose of 10 mg daily for 10 days was followed by continuous low-dose melphalan (2.5–5 mg daily), and resulted in marked clinical improvement after 8 months.

Harris *et al.*[34] reported good results with continuous, low-dose melphalan. Of seven patients given 1–4 mg daily, six improved, and the results in four were described as excellent. This regime was found to be superior to high-dose, intermittent, cyclic therapy which two patients had received. Improvement was generally seen within 3 months. One patient required only 4 months' treatment and continued to improve after melphalan was discontinued. Alterations in the levels of paraprotein were variable, and did not necessarily reflect clinical improvement. Cytotoxic therapy is not without risk, however: patients must be closely monitored by means of regular blood counts and treatment should be interrupted or stopped if there is evidence of bone marrow suppression. Although in this series the incidence of side-effects was generally low, one patient died of myelomonocytic leukaemia after 10 years of continuous therapy[34].

In contrast to a low-dose, continuous regime, Wright *et al.*[5] had better results in one patient who received an intermittent, high-dose, cyclic regime of melphalan and prednisone similar to that given for myeloma. Four-day courses of 18 mg melphalan and 140 mg prednisone daily were repeated at 6-weekly intervals. This patient had nodulocystic lesions and also underwent dermabrasion with good results. Results with either a high-dose or a low-dose regime of melphalan do not appear to be uniformly good, however, and some patients fail to respond[24,28,29].

Cyclophosphamide

Cyclophosphamide is an alkylating agent related to melphalan and might, therefore, be expected to be useful in treatment. One patient given cyclophosphamide for about six months (initially 200 mg daily for 4 months, reducing to 50 mg daily for a final 7 weeks) showed striking improvement (normal skin) that was sustained 6 months after discontinuing treatment[22]. Another patient improved with 100 mg cyclophosphamide daily for 14 months, followed by 50 mg daily[26].

Other cytotoxic agents

No benefit has been shown with chlorambucil[29] or azathioprine[29,44]. Piper *et al.*[44] treated two patients with methotrexate and had equivocal results.

OTHER TREATMENTS

Radiotherapy

Although superficial X-ray treatment was of no help in one case[14], a patient who was given radiotherapy for a coincident squamous cell carcinoma on the lip noted resolution of adjacent areas of lichen myxoedematosus[1]. He was given further radiotherapy with effect. Small fields were treated sequentially, each field being given a total dose of 3000 rad. It was suggested that radiotherapy offered a good alternative to cytotoxic treatment.

One patient responded to whole-body electron-beam therapy using 3 MeV electrons in three fractions of 800 rad each (total 2400 rad)[27].

Photochemotherapy

Farr and Ive[45] recently reported a patient with scleromyxoedema who responded to oral psoralen photochemotherapy (PUVA)[45], but other patients have shown no response[17,29,33].

Plasma exchange

One patient of ours showed striking improvement following treatment with a combination of plasma exchange, cyclophosphamide and pulsed intravenous methylprednisolone[17]. This patient continues to do well on a combination of oral prednisolone and cyclophosphamide, and skin histology has returned almost entirely to normal. She had previously failed to respond to PUVA or cyclophosphamide alone. However, another patient treated by plasmapheresis (alone and in combination with azathioprine) did not respond to treatment[29].

Retinoids

Brenner and Yust[28] reported remarkable improvement in one patient within 10 days of commencing etretinate 75 mg daily[28]. This patient had shown little response to melphalan and was taking prednisone 140 mg daily when etretinate was started.

Dermabrasion

Dermabrasion has been helpful in some patients with nodulocystic lesions[5,6].

CONCLUSION

Scleromyxoedema represents a real therapeutic challenge. Evidence regarding its treatment is based mainly on individual case reports, and treatment that may have been successful in one case may be unsuccessful in another. The best chance of success probably lies with immunosuppressive agents such as melphalan or cyclophosphamide. Nevertheless, some patients have clearly responded to other approaches, such as plasma exchange, PUVA, electron-beam therapy and etretinate, and it is encouraging to find that the options available for successful management of this condition are increasing.

References

1. Hill, T.G., Crawford, J.N., and Rogers, C.C. (1976). Successful management of lichen myxedematosus. *Arch. Dermatol*, **112**, 67–9
2. Dubreuilh, W. (1906). Fibromes miliaires folliculaires: sclérodermie consécutive. *Ann. Dermatol. Syph.*, **7**, 569–73
3. Montgomery, H. and Underwood, L.J. (1953). Lichen myxedematosus (differ-

entiation from cutaneous myxedemas or mucoid states). *J. Invest. Dermatol.*, **20**,213–33
4. Gottron, H.A. (1954). Skleromyxödem (Eine eigenartige Erscheinungsform von Myxothesaurodermie.) *Arch. Dermatol. Syph.*, **199**, 71–91
5. Wright, R.C., Franco, R.S., Denton, M.D. and Blaney, D.J. (1976). Scleromyxedema. *Arch. Dermatol.*, **112**, 63–6
6. Jepsen, L.V. (1980). Two cases of scleromyxoedema. *Acta Dermatol. Venereol. (Stockholm)*, **60**, 77–9
7. McCuistion, C.H. and Schoch, Jr, E.P. (1956). Autopsy findings in lichen myxedematosus. *Arch. Dermatol.*, **74**, 259–62
8. Rudner, E.J., Mehregan, A. and Pinkus, H. (1966). Scleromyxedema. A variant of lichen myxedematosus. *Arch. Dermatol.*, **93**, 3–12
9. Shapiro, C.M., Fretzin, D. and Norris, S. (1970). Papular mucinosis. *J. Am. Med. Assoc.*, **214**, 2052–4
10. Johnson, B.L., Horowitz, I.R., Charles, C.R. and Cooper, D.L. (1973). Dermatomyositis and lichen myxedematosus: a clinical, histopathological and electron microscopic study. *Dermatologica*, **147**, 109–22
11. Harper, R.A. and Rispler, J. (1978). Lichen myxedematosus serum stimulates human skin fibroblast proliferation. *Science*, **199**, 545–7
12. Alligood, T.R., Burnett, J.W. and Raines, B.L. (1981). Scleromyxoedema associated with esophageal aperistalsis and dermal eosinophilia. *Cutis*, **28**, 60–4
13. Muldrow, M.L. and Bailin, P.L. (1983). Scleromyxedema associated with IgG lambda multiple myeloma. *Cleve. Clin Q.*, **50**, 189–95
14. Perry, H.O., Montgomery, H. and Stickney, J.M. (1960). Further observations on lichen myxedematosus. *Ann. Intern. Med.*, **53**, 955–69
15. Findlay, G.H. and Simson, I.W. (1960). Scleromyxoedema. *S. Afr. Med. J.*, **34**, 69–71
16. James, K., Fudenberg, H., Epstein, W.L. and Shuster, J. (1967). Studies on a unique diagnostic serum globulin in papular mucinosis (lichen myxedematosus). *Clin. Exp. Immunol.*, **2**, 153–66
17. Macfarlane, A.W., Davenport, A., Verbov, J.L. and Goldsmith, H.J. (1987). Scleromyxoedema. Successful treatment with plasma exchange amd immunosuppression. *Br. J. Dermatol.*, **117**, 653–7
18. McCarthy, J.T., Osserman, E., Lombardo, P.C. and Takatsuki, K. (1964). An abnormal serum globulin in lichen myxedematosus. *Arch. Dermatol.*, **89**, 446–50
19. Verbov, J.L. (1969). Scleromyxoedema - a variant of lichen myxoedematosus (papular mucinosis). *Br. J. Dermatol.*, **81**, 871–3
20. Donald, G.F., Hensley, W.J. and McGovern, V.J. (1953). Lichen myxoedematosus (papular mucinosis): a brief review of the literature and report of a case which failed to respond to ACTH and cortisone. *Australas. J. Dermatol.*, **2**, 28–34
21. Fowlkes, R.W., Blaylock, W.K. and Mullinax, F. (1967). Immunologic studies in lichen myxedematosus. *Arch. Dermatol.*, **95**, 370–4
22. Howsden, S.M., Herndon, Jr, J.H. and Freeman, R.G. (1975). Lichen myxedematosus. A dermal infiltrative disorder responsive to cyclophosphamide therapy. *Arch. Dermatol.*, **111**, 1325–30
23. Danby, F.W., Danby, C.W.E. and Pruzanski, W. (1976). Papular mucinosis with IgG (kappa) M component. *Can. Med. Assoc. J.*, **114**, 920–2

24. Lai A Fat, R.F.M., Suurmond, D., Rádl, J. and van Furth, R. (1973). Scleromyxoedema (lichen myxoedematosus) associated with a paraprotein, IgG_1 of type kappa. *Br. J. Dermatol.*, **88**, 107–16
25. Farmer, E.R., Hambrick, Jr, G.W. and Shulman, L.E. (1982). Papular mucinosis. A clinicopathologic study of four patients. *Arch. Dermatol.*, **118**, 9–13
26. Jessen, R.T., Straight, M. and Becker, L.E. (1978). Lichen myxedematosus. Treatment with cyclophosphamide. *Int. J. Dermatol.*, **17**, 833–9
27. Lowe, N.J., Dufton, P.A., Hunter, R.D. and Vickers, C.F.H. (1982). Electron-beam treatment of scleromyxoedema. *Br. J. Dermatol.*, **106**, 449–54
28. Brenner, S. and Yust, I. (1984). Treatment of scleromyxedema with etretinate. *J. Am. Acad. Dermatol.*, **10**, 295–6
29. Westheim, A.I. and Lookingbill, D.P. (1987). Plasmapheresis in a patient with scleromyxedema. *Arch Dermatol.*, **123**, 786–9
30. Rowell, N.R., Waite, A. and Scott, D.G. (1969). Multiple serum protein abnormalities in lichen myxoedematosus. *Br. J. Dermatol.*, **81**, 753–8
31. Feldman, P., Shapiro, L., Pick, A.I. and Slatkin, M.H. (1969). Scleromyxedema. A dramatic response to melphalan. *Arch. Dermatol.*, **99**, 51–6
32. Lawrence, D.A., Tye, M.J. and Liss, M. (1972). Immunochemical analysis of the basic immunoglobulin in papular mucinosis. *Immunochemistry*, **9**, 41–9
33. Penmetcha, M., Highet, A.S. and Hopkinson, J.M. (1987). Failure of PUVA in lichen myxoedematosus: acceleration of associated multiple keratoacanthomas with development of squamous carcinoma. *Clin. Exp. Dermatol.*, **12**, 220–3
34. Harris, R.B., Perry, H.O., Kyle, R.A. and Winkelmann, R.K. (1979). Treatment of scleromyxedema with melphalan. *Arch. Dermatol.*, **115**, 295–9
35. Huth, K., Ehlers, G., Knoth, W., *et al.* (1972). Lichen myxoedematosus bei Makroglobulinämie Waldenström mit Polyneuropathie und Carpaltunnel-syndrom. *Dtsch. Med. Wochenschr.*, **97**, 152–9
36. Coskey, R.J. and Mehregan, A. (1977). Papular mucinosis. *Int. J. Dermatol.*, **16**, 741–4
37. Hardie, R.A., Hunter, J.A.A., Urbaniak, S. and Habeshaw, J.A. (1979). Spontaneous resolution of lichen myxoedematosus. *Br. J. Dermatol.*, **100**, 727–30
38. Cheung, H.S., Nicoloff, J.T., Kamiel, M.B., Spolter, L. and Nimni, M.E. (1978). Stimulation of fibroblastic biosynthetic activity by serum of patients with pretibial myxedema. *J. Invest. Dermatol.*, **71**, 12–17
39. Ohta, A., Uitto, J., Oikarinen, A.I., *et al.* (1987). Paraproteinaemia in patients with scleredema. *J. Am. Acad. Dermatol.*, **16**, 96–107
40. Truhan, A.P. and Roenigk, H.H. (1986). The cutaneous mucinoses. *J. Am. Acad. Dermatol.*, **14**, 1–18
41. Proppe, A., Becker, V. and Hardmeier, T. (1969). Skleromyxödem Arndt-Gottron und Plasmacytom. *Hautarzt*, **20**, 53–9
42. Dalton, J.E., Booth, B.H., Gray, H.R. and Evans, P.V. (1961). Lichen myxedematosus (papular mucinosis). *Arch. Dermatol.*, **83**, 230–42
43. de Mauberge, J., Ledoux, M., Collart, F., *et al.* (1987). Scléromyxoedème (Arndt-Gottron). *Dermatologica*, **174**, 197–8
44. Piper, W., Hardmeier, T. and Schäfer, E. (1967). Das Skleromyxödem Arndt-Gottron: eine paraproteinämische Erkrankung. *Schweiz. Med. Wochenschr.*, **97**, 829–38
45. Farr, P.M. and Ive, F.A. (1984). PUVA treatment of scleromyxoedema. *Br. J. Dermatol.*, **110**, 347–50

INDEX

GPSR Compliance

The European Union's (EU) General Product Safety Regulation (GPSR) is a set of rules that requires consumer products to be safe and our obligations to ensure this.

If you have any concerns about our products, you can contact us on ProductSafety@springernature.com

In case Publisher is established outside the EU, the EU authorized representative is:

Springer Nature Customer Service Center GmbH
Europaplatz 3
69115 Heidelberg, Germany

Batch number: 10607224

Printed by Printforce, the Netherlands